The dream always beg
some waiting room so
large china vase. There
room, and I could se
steadily growing darke
to get home in time. I had some kind of appointment here,
but I wasn't sure what it was.

Just then one of the doors in the hallway opened slightly
and a man in white beckoned me into the next room. I
went inside, and I saw it was a dentist's office, although it
seemed very quaint and old fashioned, and there was a
strange smell around. The dentist's chair had lots of cogs
and wheels and pulleys, and the dentist told me to lie
down on it. He said he was going to fill my holes . . .

ain in the same way, I was sitting in
somewhere, on a hard bench next to a
was a skylight up at the side of the
through the skylight that it was
, and I wondered if I'd ever be able

CELESTE T. PAUL

Women's Erotic Dreams

(and what they mean)

GRAFTON BOOKS
A Division of the Collins Publishing Group

LONDON GLASGOW
TORONTO SYDNEY AUCKLAND

Grafton Books
A Division of the Collins Publishing Group
8 Grafton Street, London W1X 3LA

A Grafton UK Paperback Original 1988
9 8 7 6 5 4

A CIP catalogue record for
this book is available from
the British Library

ISBN 0-586-20141-6

Printed and bound in Great Britain by
Collins, Glasgow

Set in Sabon

Contents

Prologue
The Dreams of Fair Women

I dreamed I was dressed in a strange outfit of rusty red suede, and I was captain of an extraordinary wooden ship. We were sailing, or *gliding* rather, across a very bright sunlit bay. Apart from me the ship was crewed entirely by men. I remember feeling very happy, almost elated. The men were naked, most of them, but they all wore chains or necklaces or some pieces of golden jewelry. They were all very handsome, and they had curly sun-bleached hair that blew in the breeze.

We sailed through a kind of whitish fog or haze, and then the ship settled close to the shore. It was a wide gravelly beach, quite deserted, and I could smell land and flowers for the first time in months. A sort of gangplank was lowered, and two of the men stood on either side of it. I grasped their long dangling cocks in my hands, and swung myself down on to the shingle.

It was then that I knew I was being chased. The men were after me. They dropped over the sides of the ship and came running across the beach toward me. The trouble was that when I ran my thighs rubbed together, and the feeling turned me on. The pleasure was so intense that it slowed me down, and I knew I could never escape. I looked back and the men were very close. Their cocks were all stiff, and the wind was blowing against the holes in their cocks and making a whistling noise.

I reached the edge of the beach, and I was just about to escape into a field of yellow poppies. But the men stood where they were, and held their cocks so that they pointed in my direction, and released long whips of white sperm. These whips caught me across my back and my face, and they stung like nettles. I could taste blood. I dropped down to my knees, and buried my face in the flowers, but the whips lashed me across my back and my bottom, and one even caught me on my vagina. I put my hands down to my stomach, and I could feel it swelling. I knew I was pregnant. My stomach rose and rose and lifted me almost clear of the flowers. Suddenly I realized what was happening. I wasn't pregnant at all. I was being fucked from the *inside*.

This erotic dream, recounted by a 26-year-old woman from Dover, Delaware, is crowded with images that would never occur in a man's dream. While some erotic dreams are common to both sexes – dreams of flying, dreams of traveling, dreams of anxiety – there are countless distinctive and fascinating images that appear in the sexual dreams of women *alone*.

Reading Freud, you might have gotten the idea that women spend their nights dreaming of nothing but penises in various symbolic shapes and forms (daggers, umbrellas, loaves of French bread). But, in fact, the sexual dreams of women have a rich supply of images that have nothing to do with that ubiquitous male projection. Women are quite capable of dreaming about their own sexual identity – their femaleness, their breasts and their vaginas, their wombs and their fallopian tubes – *without* the dream including any reference to a man.

I'm explaining this because I want you to understand that women's sexual dreams are not always soft and submissive. The female sexual dream is not a kind of mental cunt, longing for a dreamlike cock (or dagger or umbrella or loaf of French bread). It is a positive and vital thought process in its own right. It is an unconscious expression of your feminine sexual powers. When you have a sexual dream, your mind is, for once, in a perfect state of women's liberation. It is telling you what you are and what you really want. And what you are is *not* just a receptacle for daggers and French loaves, and what you want is *not* unquestioning submission and obedience to a man's sexual desires. Thirty-one-year-old Liza from Washington, DC, said:

I really discovered myself as a woman through sexual dreams. I was brought up in a very patriarchal family, and I've worked almost all my life for government departments, which are also very male-oriented and patriarchal. I always saw myself as the socket for the male plug. The *negative* rather than the positive.

Then I started having dreams in which I appeared as a man. I was a soldier sometimes or a cop or something very male and aggressive like that. I knew I was a man in the dream, but at the same time I knew I was also a woman. I guess the turning point was when I dreamed I was attacking a man in a park someplace. I think it was dark, or else we were deep among the trees. The man was walking through the park and I attacked him. He tried to run but I had enormous power, and I just hurled him on to the ground as if I was the man and he was a woman. He tried to get away, but I ripped off his pants. I looked down and his cock was bare, but it wasn't a real cock — it was a kind of cunt-cock. I knew that I could rape him — that I could actually enter him.

I held him pinned against the ground. I was naked, except for stiletto shoes, and I had muscles like Tarzan. I held his hips between my thighs, and his arms against the muddy grass. I began to move my ass up and down and round and round, real slow and undulating, and somehow my clitoris slipped into a mauve-colored juicy hole in his cunt-cock, and I was able to fuck him.

When I came, in the dream, a whole lot of thick transparent stuff seemed to pour out of me, and I had the most ecstatic feeling I can ever remember. I knew it was a dream, but the pleasure was so good that it didn't matter.

I thought about that dream for days. At first, it worried me. I wondered if I was a lesbian or a bisexual. But after a few days I started dreaming again — sex dreams — and even though they were still *positive*, they were much less *aggressive*.

I remember one dream where I was lying in bed with two men. We were all very hot, and we were sweating. I made the men lie either side of me, with their cocks against my lips, and I took two cocks into my mouth at once. I guess cocksucking might seem like a submissive kind of act, but the whole thing was that I *made* them do it.

I began to realize that my dreams were telling me to do something. They were telling me to think and behave the way I was entitled to, as a woman. To stop behaving like a socket, and be a plug instead. The strength to be myself was latent there inside me, if only I could pluck up the courage to act it out for real. My dreams were telling me that I had womanly strength.

At a time like now, when many women are confused about their sexual lives and their sexual identity, erotic dreams are priceless treasure maps to their sexual selves. In fact, erotic dreams are the only way in which a woman can discover the truth about her sexual capabilities — provided she knows how to interpret them.

But what's so important about knowing yourself as a sexual individual, and how can a dream possibly help?

Well, the importance of knowing yourself is this. Much of your sexual behavior as a woman — because of social conditioning, because of physical and emotional factors — is dominated by what men expect you to be. If your husband or lover wants a particular kind of girl around him, you tend to try and be that kind of girl, even though it may not really be you. And it goes back further than that. The sexual personality you are right now has been molded by your father, by Hollywood movies, by pin-ups and TV commercials, by romantic novelettes and magazines — by every sexual idea and image that has ever convinced you that women are acquiescent objects of male sexual lust.

Now, don't get the idea that responding to a man's sexual desires or dressing and behaving in a way which will turn men on is a bad thing. It isn't. A sexual relationship is a two-way street, and a man has just as much right to his sexual desires as you have to yours.

But you will be a better lover and a more sexually creative person if you know what your sexual identity really is. Your sex life will be all the richer if you start drawing on your own strength and your own ideas, rather than if you try to live up to someone else's concept of sexual bliss.

Your erotic dreams can help you to do this because they always tell you the truth about yourself. They may seem weird and eccentric; they may be full of visual jokes and strange puns. But no matter how they wrap it up, they are giving you a direct insight into your sexual self. All you have to do is interpret the clues, and work out just what it is that your dreaming mind is trying to tell you. Said a 28-year-old New York woman:

I dreamed I was crushing coriander seeds with a pestle and mortar. I could distinctly smell the coriander in my dream. Through the door, I could see a man's bare legs, and I knew that a naked man must be sitting in my armchair. The television was switched on, and there was some programme about locking your home against intruders. I suddenly thought to myself, 'That man – he's basting.'

The pestle and mortar are very Freudian images of the phallus and the vagina, and in this dream they probably do represent a penis and a cunt. But be warned. Freud was phallus-happy, and it's a mistake to assume that everything which sticks out in your sexual dreams is a cock. It could possibly symbolize something far more complex and far more revealing. One girl told me that her analyst had interpreted her dreams of anxiety about umbrellas as a sign of penis-phobia. But it turned out that she had really been dreaming about an aunt of hers, who used to visit her when she was very young, and caress her in a sexually disturbing way. The aunt always left her umbrella in the hall stand, and when the girl saw it there, she knew the aunt had arrived. So accurate interpretation is a case of which specific umbrella and what it signifies to you as an individual, rather than generalizing that every umbrella in every dream is a phallic symbol.

The coriander seeds were another personal memory, although they could also have represented semen. They had spiced a meal that she had once cooked for the half-seen nude in the next room, one of her past lovers. She had been worried that she hadn't been giving him all the sex he wanted (locking the home against intruders), and because of that he was *basting* – a dream pun for *masturbating*.

In her waking life, this 28-year-old New York woman was unaware of why she was feeling such sexual anxiety. This erotic dream began to give her some clues. It told her more about herself and about her relationship. In conjunction with five or six more sexual dreams, it eventually helped her to face up to some of her more serious personal problems and overcome them.

As F. W. Hildebrandt wrote in 1875: 'Dreams help us to inspect those hidden depths of our existence which are mostly beyond our reach during our waking hours. Dreams bring us such refined insight into self-knowledge and such revelations of half-conscious dispositions and powers that on waking up, we may well admire the sharp-eyed demon that helped us find the hidden plot. A dream can warn us from within with the voice of a watchman stationed at the central observatory of our spiritual life. And our dreams can also warn us of the dangerous steps we have already taken!'

Every woman dreams, without exception – even women who claim that they never do. Conclusive research at Harvard, the University of Chicago, Mount Sinai Hospital, the Walter Reed Institute of Research – as well as dozens of other hospitals and institutions all over the world – has shown beyond doubt that everybody has at least *three* and sometimes as many as *nine* dreams every night.

Nobody has yet discovered just why it is that you dream. But we do know that if you don't dream for long enough, you will probably wind up psychotic. Volunteers have been deprived of dreams (by constant waking whenever electronic monitors showed dream activity in the brain) and have started, after some length of time, to behave in irrational, bizarre, and disoriented ways. For some reason, we need our dreams.

As you sleep, your brain and body go through recurrent 90-minute curves of deep and shallow sleep. You have your weirdest (and unfortunately your most forgettable) dreams when you're in deep sleep just after midnight. But your most vivid and memorable dreams occur during REM sleep. REM stands for Rapid Eye Movement, and scientists have labeled this particular kind of sleep in this way because your eyes flicker back and forth under your eyelids as though you're looking at images inside your mind.

During REM dreaming, men frequently have erections. That's why men often awake with a hard-on – it's a left-over from their last REM dream. Some grateful wives of older men call it the *morning glory*, and it just goes to show that you have something to thank dreams for. But there is no research that shows whether or not women experience arousal of the clitoris during REM dreams. From limited personal checks, it seems to me that they do, but it's time some laboratory had a look into it. Here's the sexual dream of a 25-year-old New York fashion designer:

I dreamed I was working as an artist in a very hot jungle someplace. We heard drums and we knew there was danger. We managed to get back to our airplane, which was hidden by leaves and creepers. Inside, it was humid, and there were several journalists sitting at tables and typing. But in the back of the plane, three or four girls and men were having an orgy. Their bodies were sweating and all knotted up together. I could see gaping vaginas and asses, and I had a sudden urge to plunge my tongue between some girl's legs. After all, I thought, they're all so tangled up that they won't know that it's me . . . I woke up, and I was very sexually excited. I had to masturbate to get back to sleep.

Throughout history women's sexual dreams have been considered important, and there have been many attempts to interpret them. In the Cairo Museum, there is ancient Egyptian papyrus which explains the sexual dreams of women as follows: 'If a woman kisses her husband, she will have trouble; if a horse couples with her, she will be violent with her husband; if an ass couples with her, she will be punished for great fault; if a goat couples with her, she will die promptly; if a ram couples with her, Pharaoh will be full of kindness to her; if a Syrian couples with her, she will weep, for she will let a slave couple with her; if she gives birth to a cat, she will have many children; if she gives birth to a dog, she will have a boy; if she gives birth to an ass, she will have an idiot child; if she gives birth to a crocodile, she will have many children.'

The Assyrians and the Babylonians also had a rich dream lore, and there are ancient dream books from the Hebrew, Siamese, Arabic, French, Italian, Chinese, German, and Russian cultures. They all interpret dreams in different ways, but usually the accuracy of their interpretations is not improved by their insistence on seeing every image in a woman's sexual dream as a symbol of something else. A woman couldn't have a dream about cooking noodles without it meaning that she was going to have a happy and prosperous sexual affair; she couldn't dream about a broken knife without it meaning that she was going to be unlucky in love; and she couldn't dream about rubies, squeezed lemons, or pencils without being assured that she was going to be passionately in love, hard up for money, and lucky with her lover.

Some of the old dream books are still worth going back to, even today. One of the best was that of Artemidorus, the *Oneirocritica*, written nearly 1,800 years ago. He came up with some reasonably canny remarks, such as, 'All monsters and impossibilities are vain hopes of things that will not happen,' and 'To fly is to be lifted above those about one.' By 1880 the English-language edition of the

Oneirocritica had run into thirty-two reprints. But since then, there have been dozens and dozens of 'dream dictionaries', most of which are a hotchpotch of ancient dream interpretations, astrology, half-baked Freudian psychology, and sheer uninformed guesswork. If you start looking into any of those for interpretations of your erotic dreams, you're liable to come up with some pretty contradictory and peculiar suggestions.

If I check four of them at random, for example, I find that a sexual dream about cows can either be interpreted as conflict with your mother, hard work without much fun, good luck and prosperity, or anxiety about sexual discontent. Take your pick.

We don't find that modern psychoanalysts always do better than the occult interpreters of dreams, either. In his book, *The Clinical Use of Dreams*, Dr Walter Bonime tells how a significant dream of one of his women patients had been dismissed out of hand by her previous analyst, and how the interpretation had confused and distressed her. She had dreamed that she was walking down a long corridor with closed doors on each side, and as she stepped along the shabby carpet, she could hear behind each of the doors laughter and chatter, which made her feel lonesome and neglected. Her analyst had said that the corridor was her vagina, and that she felt sexually ignored.

'His interpretation was a shock to me,' said the woman. 'There was nothing in it I recognized. I felt that there was more in the dream, and I was losing the value of the dream somehow.' Nine years after she had had the dream, she told Bonime that she was convinced the dream really meant that she felt hopeless about her marriage. 'If I had understood the dream and consciously recognized how hopeless I felt about my marriage, I would have taken steps to get out of it at the time, instead of waiting five more long, miserable years.'

This is exactly the point I made earlier on. The 'vagina interpretation' was a man's concept of a woman's dream, and it was wrong. It was also wrong of the analyst to give his patient a totally dogmatic and unbending interpretation of what she was supposed to be dreaming about when she knew in herself that it wasn't right.

Freud and his followers believed that the images in dreams are symbols and disguises, and that every dream was a complicated coded message to be decoded by the analyst. All projections were phallic symbols, all holes and tunnels (and corridors) were vaginal symbols, and so on.

Jung, the Swiss psychoanalyst who broke away from Freud to develop a much more flexible therapy, said that the disguises were too complicated to be believable. In the Talmud, he reminded Freud, it says, 'the dream is its own interpretation.' And Jung said 'the dream is a natural event, and there is no reason under the sun why we should assume that it is a crafty device to lead us astray.' Dr H. G. Baynes, one of Jung's followers, said that to think of dreams as disguises was like an English visitor going to Paris and assuming that the Parisians were talking gibberish just to make him look a fool!

Later on, we'll take a look at some of Freud and Jung's theories as well as some much newer ideas about dream interpretation, but right now it's worth making the point that the most important interpreter of your erotic dreams is *you*.

Professor Calvin S. Hall of the University of California at Santa Cruz, author of *The Meaning of Dreams*, says this:

One does not dream in order to provide psychologists with information about the mind or human nature. Nor do we have dreams in order to recall them in the morning, to tell them to our friends, or to our psychoanalyst. They are not messages or omens or prophecies; they are not the experiences of a disembodied soul; they are not the movements of the eyeballs; they are not the guardians or sentinels of sleep; and they do not reduce tension by fulfilling wishes. They exist for their own reasons, whatever those reasons may be. But because they do exist, we can utilize them advantageously in exploring the contents of the mind ... Dreams may not always be a reliable indication of how a person may act when awake, but they can be depended upon to reveal the underlying motivation for the person's behavior, often in a crude yet unmistakable form.

Dr Ann Faraday, the British dream expert, supports this view: '... psychoanalysts have done us a disservice by associating dream interpretation with mental illness and spreading the idea that any form of self-therapy which involves "probing the depths" is a dangerous business. While it is true that there are disturbed people who cannot cope with life without expert therapeutic help, there are also millions of other intelligent and basically "normal" people who are perfectly capable of exploring their own dreams for greater self-knowledge.'

Self-knowledge is what this book is all about. It tells you how you dream, why you dream, and how to interpret your own dreams. Even more, it tells you how to use your dreams in your own sexual relationships and sexual life, so that you can actively improve your daytime erotic activities by what you learn from your sleep.

As G. Bachelard wrote in his book *La Terre et les Rêveries de la Volonté*: 'the most productive decisions are associated with nocturnal dreams. The man (or woman) who sleeps badly cannot have confidence in himself. In fact, sleep, which is held to be an interruption of the consciousness, links us to ourselves. The normal dream, the true dream, is thus often the prelude, and by no means the sequel, to our active life.'

In other words, your sexual dreams can become an integral part of discovering yourself and improving your sexual talents and sexual techniques. Contrary to popular myth (mainly based on Freudian misconceptions), our dreams do not try to hide our real sexual personality from ourselves, and a whole storehouse of erotic riches is waiting there for you to sift and interpret. Once you have the knack of reasonably accurate self-analysis, you'll find that most sexual dreams are very lucid and easy to divine.

Some erotic dreams are completely blatant. Dr Ann Faraday says that she once woke a male student in the middle of a REM dream, and he was most annoyed with her because he was having a very stimulating dream about making love to his mother. 'I myself had several lovely dreams of my brother making love to me from behind,' she says, 'and was very cross to be awakened from them by the alarm clock.'

Sexual dreams were thought by Freud to be a safety-valve – a way of quenching forbidden desires by playing them out in the mind. But modern research shows that there is no evidence that dreams about sex will satisfy you. If anything, they may even have the reverse effect by bringing out into the open desires that you didn't previously recognize that you had. Dr Faraday says that after dreaming about sex with her brother, she now finds herself far more incestuously attracted to him than she ever was before.

Other sexual dreams *feel* erotic when you're actually having them, but on retrospect seem extraordinarily non-sexual. That's because the images are freewheeling their way through your dreaming mind, and you're thinking at random without assembling your ideas into the neat, logical patterns that your waking mind usually imposes. Your brain is *always* a constant babble of puns, associations, jokes, images, recollections, and anecdotes – but normally you suppress the background chatter and select the cool, calm logic. When you're dreaming, however, that often doesn't happen, and you end up with something like this dream from one of Dr Faraday's colleagues:

> As I was drifting off to sleep, I saw those colored balls of this afternoon's film *rolling* towards me. This led me to think of chocolate *rolls* and of woman's *role* in society. It was, of course, to *roll* her hips, and I immediately found H. standing before me in the dream *rolling* her hips in a very seductive manner. This led me straight into a sex dream about her.

Although dreams like these may seem nonsensical, it is very important for you as a woman to take the trouble to see the truth behind the nonsense. As Professor Hall says: 'The truth revealed in dreams is the same truth we have to face and deal with in waking life. How we deal with that truth while we are asleep and dreaming is not in itself important. How we deal with it during waking life is of the greatest importance to our personal well-being and to the well-being of society.'

At this time, one of the most essential ingredients of a woman's personal well-being is a fulfillment of her sexual potential. From her erotic dreams, she can find the sexual being that she really is. Germaine Greer made the point that women are unfitted for the sexual participation they have so far been offered, but many are not capable of running their own lives because they have so successfully been conditioned into being dependent. She says:

> Most psychologists are still bred in the expectation that a woman's sexuality becomes feminine only when it declines into passivity. But physiologically it's not true. The sexuality of the adolescent girl is not male – it's hers, it's female. What happens when she's grown up is that she's taught a sex role. If she cannot adapt to it she is branded as a neurotic, a fixate, a lesbian if you like.
> Women are actually taught that normality is passivity. The belief that the man fucks the woman has led to a fact. The man *does* fuck the woman most of the time, because the woman

doesn't know that there's anything for her to do but lie back and take it. She knows that sometimes she's got to do a bit of moaning and heaving just so he'll feel good and won't feel too lonely up there, but she doesn't know much more than that. Yet men and women are geared to different sexual rhythms and responses. Nothing in life is necessarily so. We can change it all. We can even change menstrual patterns.

The way men and women behave now is inevitably due to their inheritance of conditioning. But it's also contingent, because it is dependent on inheritance of conditioning, so it can be changed. And it better be.

There is no more effective way for you to change your life as a woman for the better than by exploring your sexual dreams. Professor Hall notes that 'the dynamics of dreams are also the dynamics of society. Consequently, when we are studying dreams, we are not only studying the individual but we are also studying his social behavior and the institutes he creates.' In other words, your sexual dreams will reveal to you where you believe you stand in relation to men, in relation to other women, in relation to sexual desires and sexual variations. Out of the mass of information about yourself that your dreams will give you, you will be able to construct a profile of yourself that will be as near to the true you as any kind of assessment could ever get.

What's more, your sexual dreams will also tell you what you really want out of sex. *Desires* that you may be afraid to admit to yourself when you're awake. *Fantasies* that you've suppressed because you don't think they're quite the kind of thing that a lady ought to be thinking about. *Lusts* that always seemed embarrassing.

And once you know what you are and what you want, your dreams will also be able to tell you whether you have the basic initiative and drive to be able to satisfy those desires, fantasies, and lusts. A 25-year-old Boston steno-grapher said:

I always thought there was something wrong with me, that I was oversexed. My parents used to be so puritanical, and they frowned on sex so much that I began to believe that it was rude and dirty, and that making love was on the same kind of level as going to the bathroom. You did it because you had to do it, but you didn't actually *enjoy* it.

I was always having dreams about sex, but mostly I put them out of my mind and forgot them, because I felt guilty about them. But there was one dream that I had over and over again all through the summer, and it got so persistent that I couldn't ignore it.

The dream always began in the same way. I was sitting in some waiting room somewhere, on a hard bench next to a large china vase. There was a skylight up at the side of the room, and I could see through the skylight that it was steadily growing darker, and I wondered if I'd ever be able to get home in time. I had some kind of appointment here, but I wasn't sure what it was.

Just then one of the doors in the hallway opened slightly, and a man in white beckoned me into the next room. I went inside, and I saw it was a dentist's office, although it seemed to be very quaint and old-fashioned, and there was a strange smell around. I thought the smell was like 'antique oranges'. The dentist's chair had lots of cogs and wheels and pulleys, and the dentist told me to lie down on it. He said he was going to fill my holes.

The dentist's nurse appeared. She was wearing a white starched cap, and she was wearing one of those black bras that leave most of your breasts bare. She had enormous breasts, the biggest breasts that I'd ever seen in my whole life, and the nipples were huge and stiff and very red. I thought that she must use lipstick on them, and I was going to ask if she did, but I had to lie on the couch just then, and the dentist put something like a hard purple plum into my mouth and told me to suck on it.

The nurse was also wearing black stockings and suspenders, and very high stiletto shoes. I looked down between her legs, and her pubic hair was very long and shiny, and she had tied it up with red ribbons. I knew there was something hiding between her legs. Perhaps it was a tongue that came out of her cunt, but I couldn't be sure.

The dentist and the nurse made me lie right back. The lights were very bright, and they made me open my legs wide apart. Then they locked my legs apart with clamps, and cut open my panties with something that looked like a pair of curling tongs.

I said to them: 'What are you doing?' but they simply smiled and nodded and that was all. Then they brought down a kind of shiny chrome and steel apparatus that had a big boss-like metal cylinder. They lined up the cylinder between my legs, and then the dentist pulled a lever and there was a hiss like the brakes of a truck, and the cylinder was forced straight up me. I could actually look down between my legs and see this huge shiny thing, and the red lips of my cunt clinging around it.

The dentist leaned over me and said: 'How does it feel?' I said: 'I think you've damaged me. I think I'm dying. I shouldn't have done this.' All he said was: 'That's all right, my dear. We'll be able to put the plants in later.'

Suddenly I was waiting for a train. I was standing on the subway platform and I knew that a train was coming. I thought to myself: 'Now I know what they were trying to do to me. They want to fuck me with a train.' And that's when I usually woke up, or else the dream ended and I started dreaming about something else.

In a later chapter we'll see just how the images and events of erotic dreams like this can be interpreted in detail – and how, if the girl had only understood the most pressing message of the dream, she could have helped herself to discover more about sex and balance her sexual attitudes.

But right now, it's sufficient to say that dreams like these do have a distinct capacity for helping you to solve your problems. Dr Faraday recalls dreams in which she was being beheaded. These occurred at a time in her life when she was developing her intellect at the expense of her emotions, and it was only when she took a more balanced view of life that the dreams ceased.

Jung believed that dreams are part of an inner drive within the mind to keep itself healthy and integrated and so steadily develop itself towards maturity. Dreams are like the lymph which forms scabs over cuts in the skin or the organisms within your bloodstream which fight disease. They are part of the process of being yourself and realizing your self's potential.

Dr Faraday reports the dream of a girl who pictured herself wandering around a hospital trying to procure an abortion because she was pregnant by an animal. In her dream, she was trying to puzzle out what kind of an animal it was going to be. She recalled that she had slept in stables on occasions, and once as a child she had taken her pet rat to bed with her.

The possible explanation for this dream, suggests Dr Faraday, is that the girl, who was fairly liberal minded, was trying at the time to decide whether to sleep with a Negro student or not. Although racial prejudice was totally alien to her conscious mind, her unconscious mind saw the Negro as an 'animal'. There is relentless truthfulness in dreams.

But once you can understand the meaning of a sexual dream like that, you can make a much clearer decision about what you're going to do. Dr Faraday doesn't tell us whether the girl ever slept with her black beau or not. But if she did, she would at least have been forewarned about possible problems in the relationship – problems which her waking mind might never have admitted 'out loud'.

Your dreams almost always deal with *current* problems, *current* situations. They may be crowded with symbols that are derived from way back in your memory, but few modern dream researchers agree with Freud that they are reflections of your childhood desires and impulses.

A major key to understanding your dreams is to look at your current problems and think: 'What difficulty am I trying to sort out right now about which this dream has exactly the *opposite* viewpoint from me?' You see, dreams tend to balance out your unconscious opinions against your conscious opinions. And just like the girl student dreamed of being pregnant by an animal, when she really thought she liked her Negro pal, so you might be dreaming something obscure and peculiar that it telling you what you genuinely think about one of your daytime problems.

Another example from a friend of mine: She dreamed she was having intercourse with her father, whom she usually hated. Only when she thought more deeply about her dream did she begin to understand that maybe she loved her father rather a lot. Even sexually. Her conscious mind was only reacting to him with hatred because she didn't want to admit she had feelings that 'normal' girls weren't supposed to have.

Apart from establishing your identity as a woman and apart from assisting you to solve your sexual problems, dreams can do something else for you. They can help you develop better sexual techniques and more satisfying (not to mention more regular) orgasms. This isn't at all as far-fetched as it might seem. Orgasm failure is by far the most common female sex problem. Some sexologists report enquiries from over sixty percent of women patients about orgasm difficulty. Most of these failures are caused by psychological blocks of one kind or another. Often, you're not consciously aware of what it is that prevents you from reaching satisfactory climaxes. But the answer is someplace inside you, and it could well be revealed by your sexual dreams. As Professor Hall remarks: 'The prevalence of sex dreams, the nature of the sexual activities, and one's sexual partners will reveal interesting information about the dreamer's sexual feelings and orientation.'

To show just how precisely your erotic dreams can reflect your sexual activities, Professor Hall cites the case of Marie. Sexually promiscuous when she was in her twenties, Marie kept a dream diary then and also when she was in her sixties. Although there was almost forty years between the diaries, it was plain that the contents of her sexual dreams had hardly altered in all that time. There were the same number of males and females, the same types of objects, the same number of friendly and aggressive interactions between herself and the characters in her dreams. The only notable differences were that, when she was in her twenties, she dreamed more about being a victim of male sexual aggression, and when she was in her sixties, she dreamed more about sex with strangers. Both of these changes reflected with great accuracy the subtle changes that had occurred in her waking life. As she had grown older, she had gained more confidence (hence she dreamed less about being a victim of male aggression), and she had also lost many of her close friends (hence she dreamed more about strangers).

Here's a dream from a 19-year-old Minneapolis girl which shows how concisely and clearly an erotic dream can present the facts of your current worries:

I dreamed I was sitting in the center of the city, on a bench, and it was a hot day in September. The leaves were falling from the trees, but this didn't seem strange, even though they were all crisp and curled up. I was wearing a short cotton dress, and I knew that I didn't have any panties on underneath. I was reading a book. It was a thick book, with very creamy pages. I remember thinking that this kind of paper was called 'cream-laid'. The book had extremely erotic illustrations in it. I can't describe them now, because they weren't actually erotic in the sense that they showed penises or vaginas or anything like that, but they had a kind of forbiddenness about them that turned me on.

I lifted my heels on to the bench, and I opened my legs up and started to masturbate. I can remember pushing almost my whole hand into my vagina, and the sucking noise that it made when I pushed it in and out. I was very excited, very sexually excited, and I pulled my dress up even further and started caressing my own breasts and nipples, and tugging my nipples out two or three inches.

Just then, my father came up. He was dressed in a very badly fitting suit that looked as though he'd kept it since the 1930s. He looked angry and asked me what I was doing. I said I was only looking at pictures of naked people, and that naked people weren't anything to get worked up about. I tried to hide the fact that I was masturbating by laying the book over my legs, but I kept on doing it. It didn't occur to me to stop.

My mother came past with a basketful of shopping. She called out to my father: 'Leave the girl alone. She has to learn.' My father took his penis out. It looked pale and fat. He brought it over to where I was sitting, and said: 'Well, if you want a bite of it, it tastes like caramel candy.'

Although the appearance in your sexual dreams of anyone you know is no guarantee that you're really dreaming about them, your mother and your father are usually exactly who they appear to be. This dream was a summing-up of a problem that this 19-year-old girl had been facing in her waking life. Her father was repressive about sex and did not like to discuss it in front of her or even give her reasonable information about birth control or dating. Her mother, however, was far more understanding and lenient and encouraged her to find out about sex for herself. For me, though, the most fascinating part of this dream is the last few moments, when her father suddenly offers her his penis to bite. The girl herself thought this might mean that her father was repressive about sex because he was secretly attracted to her — until I pointed out that your dreams are entirely the creation of your *own* mind and can't let you in on anything that you don't have any way of knowing about, such as the secret thoughts of other people. The bite sequence could mean that during waking hours she had sensed that her father was attracted to her. But it was more likely that she felt sexually curious about him, as a man. When she found a regular boyfriend, sex dreams about her father would probably fade away.

There was a wealth of detail in this dream that gave the girl clues about her sexual interests, her sexual attitudes, and her real state of mind. Dreams are marvelously clear in the way they make particular points — like the 1930s suit that indicated how old-fashioned she thought her father was. Like the 'cream-laid' paper, a double-pun on two words of sexual slang. Like the falling leaves, a common dream image for passing time. There were other things, like the tugging of her nipples, which only the girl herself was able to understand and interpret.

Before you start to interpret your own sexual dreams, it's worth clearing away any of the myths and misconceptions that you might have about dreaming and what you can expect to learn from it. I've always found that one of the greatest obstacles in sexual dream interpretation is a vague acquaintance with the theories of Freud. Now, it's certainly true that in some erotic dreams, penises are disguised as pointed objects, and vaginas are disguised as hollow objects, but you cannot automatically assume that this is so until you have tried to understand what the objects really mean to you. Don't try to impose a sexual meaning on a dream that doesn't seem to have any sexual connotations or sexual feelings attached to it, or you'll wind up even more confused than when you started.

But remember too that all dreams have some kind of reason or purpose, and that reason or purpose is concerned with your identity as a person and as a woman. Erica Jong recalls a spate of dreams 'full of elevators, platforms in space, enormously steep and slippery staircases, ziggurat temples I had to climb, mountains, towers, ruins . . . I had the sense that I was *assigning* myself dreams as some sort of cure.'

Beware, too, of identifying archetypal characters in your sexual dreams too swiftly. Many sexual dreams feature policemen, princesses, queens, demons, and other stock figures. Jung believed that these characters, and other universal symbols such as circles and snakes and crosses, all come from a collective unconscious. In other words, there is a deep-down level in all of our minds where we all share the same images and ideas. He pointed out in substantiation of this theory that the myths and legends of many different countries bear remarkable and unexplained similarities, and that even his nonreligious patients had dreams about angels and devils and divine heroes. If you cannot readily identify some of the characters in your dreams, Jung suggested that you should see if they relate to any of the archetypes. Instead of representing real people, they might represent abstract ideas like authority or aggression or lust or temptation.

One of Dr Faraday's subjects, an ultrarespectable young lady, had dreams of being followed by a gypsy girl, who would mischievously make her fall over cliffs or into rivers. When the subject was unable to identify who this gypsy might be, Dr Faraday suggested that she possibly represented a hidden waywardness in the subject's personality – a dark side of herself. She was using Jung's idea that we all have a 'shadow' – an archetypal devil who haunts us, and who represents the feelings and desires we normally repress.

There is no evidence that your dreams can predict the future, although several clairvoyantes claim that they can. I prefer to stick to Jung's point of view that dreams can present you with *possibilities* for the future based on available evidence. Since your unconscious mind may be in possession of more evidence than your conscious mind, it could be that the possibilities seem almost magically lucid.

Don't dismiss any dreams because they seem insignificant. I was amazed to read in a comparatively recent book, *The Dreamer's Dictionary* by Stearn Robinson and Tom Corbett, the solemn adjunct to 'make sure that the dream is potentially a prophetic one and not merely of the digestive or "cheese" variety.' Your dreams are much more interesting than mystic warnings or astrological predictions. They tell you about yourself, and not about events or actions which you have played no part in bringing about. Compared to the discovery of your sexual potential, dreams about winning a fortune on the Kentucky Derby or about Otis Redding crashing into Lake Mendota are pretty small potatoes.

Sex and aggression are claimed by some theorists to be the two principal motivating forces of society. While you might argue about this concept as far as waking life is concerned, it is indisputably true about dream life. But up until now, few dream studies have drawn distinctions between the sexual and aggressive dreams of men and the sexual and aggressive dreams of women.

Women see themselves as the victims of aggression far more often than men. Their sexual dreams are also much more preoccupied with problems of social morality and marriage, not to mention birth and pregnancy. While men may dream about having children, their dream offspring will usually appear at a convenient age, already walking and talking, whereas women dream about the baby actually emerging from their bodies. There are dozens of other differences, and we shall explore these as we enter the strange, wild, but often beautiful world of women's sexual dreams.

It is sometimes said that the Empress Wu Hu, a sexually oriented Oriental of the T'ang Dynasty, had a dream in which she was the keeper of a garden of exquisite flowers. Men traveled from many far lands to admire her flowers, and with one flower in particular they fell in love and begged her to let them kiss it. From that dream, she is said to have devised her very personal concept of royal homage, in which she made visiting ambassadors and dignitaries kneel before her and lick her vulva.

Maybe you won't have such royal treatment after you've discovered the meanings of your sexual dreams. But this could be the starting point for pleasures that, up until now, you've only dreamed about.

BOOK ONE
Discovering Your Erotic Dreams

1

What Women Dream About

I was the bride at a wonderful wedding. It was taking place in a huge lofty cathedral, and there were choirs singing and thousands of guests, and the floor was thick with pink blossom. I was walking up the aisle and my bridegroom was walking next to me. I knew without being told that he was Clark Gable's younger brother Abel. I knew that Clark Gable was dead, but Abel Gable looked exactly like him – in fact, *was* him – so it didn't matter.

They were reading the marriage ceremony, but it seemed to be very windy, and people kept leaving the cathedral until there were hardly any guests left at all. The hymn books were blowing about, and the blossom was flying through the air, and we all had to shout to make ourselves heard. The next thing I knew, my wedding dress was being blown away, and I was standing there naked except for my tights.

Clark Gable or his brother or whoever it was turned around and looked at me, and said, 'We'd better consummate the marriage on the organ,' and he lifted me up in his arms and carried me through a curtain and across to a kind of barrel-organ that was standing in the corner of the room. As he carried me, his fingers went up into my pussy, and he waggled them around and smiled. It gave me a nice feeling between my legs, but I wasn't sure that I loved him anymore.

He laid me down on the floor next to the organ, and he took off his pants. It was still windy and his shirttails flapped. For some reason he had to keep on winding the handle of the barrel-organ while we had sex, and I thought this was ridiculous, but I knew that I would have to put up with it, because it was absolutely necessary if we wanted to have children.

He had an enormous penis. It must have been three feet long, and it felt very hard and rather warm, like a piece of polished wood that you've been holding in your hand for a long time. He said it would have to go into my bottom, up through my intestines, then out of my mouth, round again and into my pussy, otherwise it would be too long for me. I didn't like the sound of that at all, and I started to argue and struggle. But he forced me back against the floor, and he tangled my wrists up in the spokes of the wheels of the barrel-organ. I tried to get free, but it was impossible. My breasts seemed to have grown enormously, and they were so huge and heavy that they hung down on either side of my chest.

Clark Gable lifted my bottom off the cold, dusty floor, and he forced my thighs apart until they cracked. He pressed his enormous penis up against my bottom-hole, and began to force it inside me. I thought it was going to hurt, but surprisingly it didn't. In fact, the more my bottom-hole was stretched, the nicer the feeling started to grow, and soon I was saying mmmm-mmmm-mmmm, and wriggling my hips around to help him force his penis in faster.

I could feel his penis sliding right up inside me, and before I knew what was going on, it was coming out of my throat, and sliding out of my mouth. I could look down and see it sticking out from between my lips like a fat red tongue. I pulled it further and further out of my mouth, then down between my legs, and I fed it up into my pussy.

There was strange music somewhere, and the sound of it made me even more excited. I knew I was going to have some incredible new kind of orgasm. A *locust*-orgasm. There was something about the music that reminded me of locusts, rubbing their legs together. I said to my lover: 'Are you going to give me your sperm, darling?' and he leaned over me like a balloon. His face seemed swollen and airy, as though it wasn't attached to anything. He was holding a silver spoon in each hand, and he carefully poured warm sperm from each one into my eyes. I closed my eyes and let the sperm run out of the corners of my eyes, and then I had a strange orgasm that made me feel as if I was dying. I woke up, and I can remember thinking: 'Well I may be dead, but at least I've had sex with Clark Gable.'

This – the erotic dream of a 22-year-old secretary from Washington, DC – contains some of the most powerful images that women conjure up in their sexual dreams. Marriage, celebrities, rape, child-bearing and orgasm. There are also fascinating individual variations, however – like the way in which 'Clark Gable's' penis emerges from her mouth, and is then used by the dreamer herself to make love to herself. Could this be love, or could it be masturbation? And why the silver spoons and the warm sperm poured into the eyes?

There have been several attempts to record the contents of women's sexual dreams. Havelock Ellis and Kinsey both had a go, and Kinsey's statistics, although they are now twenty years out of date, make some interesting points. Let's take Kinsey's figures for the dreams of sexually *experienced* women, for example. Thirty-nine percent of them had dreams about intercourse which actually brought them to orgasm; the same percentage had orgasmic dreams of other kinds of sex contact with men; but only one percent reached orgasm with dreams about making love to animals, being pregnant or giving birth, or being involved in sadomasochistic situations.

In dreams which did *not* provoke orgasms, thirty percent of sexually experienced women dreamed about intercourse, but only four percent dreamed of rape, and less than two percent dreamed of sadomasochism or bestiality (sex with animals).

Sexually *inexperienced* women showed slightly different dream patterns. In dreams that brought them to orgasm, ten percent dreamed of intercourse and seven percent dreamed of lesbian love. Two percent dreamed of pregnancy and childbirth, and only one percent of petting and sadomasochistic experiences. In dreams that didn't bring them to orgasm, Kinsey's inexperienced ladies reported thirty-six percent for dreams of intercourse, sixteen percent for lesbian contact, about the same as the experienced ladies (four percent) for rape, and for sadomasochism and bestiality (two percent).

One or two commentators have concluded that these figures show how little connection there is between women's sexual dreams and their real-life sexual experience. But all they actually show is that *of remembered dreams,* more are probably concerned with plain old sexual intercourse than with deviations and kinks. Since we don't ever remember more than a fraction of our dreams, and we conveniently tend to suppress those dreams which embarrass our waking conscience, Kinsey's statistics can never amount to more than a very rough guide. Remember, too, that they were assembled in the 1950s, when women were more sexually repressed than they are today.

Women's sexual dreams vary from men's sexual dreams in several fascinating ways. For instance, recent statistics show that women dream of being at home in familiar surroundings more than men do, and that they dream of being indoors more often than men. Men dream about other men more often than they do about women – about two men to one woman. But women dream about men and women in equal proportions.

Women dream more frequently about female relatives than they do about male relatives. They also dream more about female friends than male friends. Men, understandably, dream more about male friends and relatives. But both men and women dream more about male strangers than female strangers.

The overall indication is that women are slightly more interested in their dreams with other women, but men are far more interested in other men.

Another notable difference is in the type of celebrity who appears in male and female dreams. Studies seem to suggest that women dream primarily about entertainers and film stars, while men dream primarily about politicians and intellectuals.

Men are more physically aggressive in their dreams, whereas women are more argumentative and verbally aggressive. Women are equally aggressive and equally friendly towards men and women, but when they're aggressive towards a man, they are much more aggressive than they would be with a woman. The same goes for friendliness. Women dream about being sexually attacked by men far more often than men dream about attacks from women, sexual or otherwise.

In comparison with men, women dream less of physical activity, less of success and failure, much more of emotion, less of size, more of color.

In all, it's clear that women's sexual dreams are dealing with different sexual situations in different terms and with different ideals in mind. There are obviously many symbols and images that apply equally to male and female sex dreams, but if we want to be really accurate about you and your problems, then we have to analyze female dreams in completely female ways. As women are becoming increasingly aware of their sexual and social rights, the stuff of female erotic dreams is inevitably growing further and further away from the stuff of male erotic dreams, and with every advance in women's liberation it will need to be analyzed with greater attention to women's changing role. A woman who is trying to find out why she has trouble with her orgasm is not going to have dreams about tripping through the meadows in a picture hat, with her poet-lover at her heels.

I dreamed I was driving my husband's car through Georgia in the pouring rain. It wasn't night, but it was very dark. I tried to drive around some very difficult bends, but something made a grinding sound under the hood, and the car stopped. I had to climb out, open the hood, and try to find out what was wrong. I was wearing a dishtowel around my waist, and apart from that I was completely nude. The rain soaked the towel, and it started to slide down. I kept trying to hitch it up, but it slid down even more, and I knew that in a few seconds I would end up stark naked.

It was dark under the car's hood, and I could only work by feel. I suddenly discovered that instead of an engine, there was a man lying under the hood, on his back, with his legs kind of tucked underneath him. I was fumbling around to find the engine, and I kept touching his body. His balls and his cock. I kept apologizing, but he didn't say anything, and I knew it was my husband. I thought to myself that I must find a way of sorting this mechanical problem out, or my husband would never forgive me. I reached inside the hood again and began to pull my husband's cock up and down.

I was aware of another man standing behind me. He held my waist in his hands, and he opened my legs with his knee, and while I was massaging my husband inside the car, he pressed himself up behind me and started having intercourse with me. I couldn't see him, but I could feel him. He had a strange cock that seemed to twist and vibrate inside me. I suddenly understood that this was the way to get over my mechanical problems. If I had somebody to do this to me while I tried to repair the car, everything would be all right. It seemed so obvious that I couldn't think why it hadn't come to me before.

The next thing I knew, I was home again. My sister was there, and she was carrying a small cake. She asked where my husband was, and I opened the hood of the car. But there was nothing inside there at all, except an engine. I looked at the car again, and my husband was sitting in the back seat. I rushed over to tell him that I knew what the problem was, but he closed the window of the car, and we couldn't hear each other speak. My sister said: 'It's all over now, then?'

This was the erotic dream of a 29-year-old housewife from Meade, Maryland. It didn't take much self-analysis to work out what she was dreaming about. She had been having difficulty reaching an orgasm for years, and she had always told herself that it was *her* fault, and that her husband's sexual technique was not to blame. The dream, however, said different and even offered a couple of alternatives. Either an extramarital lover or a vibrator. The cake was a symbol of her sister's domesticity and married bliss, which she had always envied. The car was a fairly archetypal phallic image, particularly since her naked husband was under the hood, and the setting, she later realized, came from the simple fact that she had *A Rainy Night in Georgia* on the brain.

The things that women dream about vary enormously according to their personality and their problems. But the most common sexual dreams appear to be these: dreams of rape, of marriage and home, of birth and pregnancy, of nudity in public, of celebrities, of orgasm, of incest, of sadomasochism and bestiality, of lesbianism, and last, but not at all least, of sexual freedom.

There are no reliable figures to tell us just what percentage of dreams is about which topic, and as we've already seen from Kinsey's statistics, they wouldn't tell us very much anyway. Whether you recall a dream or not depends on whether you wake up quickly or slowly, whether you're tired or not-so-tired, whether you feel like making the effort to remember it, and whether you're the kind of person who's interested in recalling dreams. Women report their dreams with varying degrees of accuracy, too. The waking mind often imposes an order and a logical sequence on to dreams that was never there in the first place. And dreamers will often try to analyze their dreams as they write them down, which can frequently destroy the dream's validity.

It strikes me very forcibly that most women's sexual dreams are dreams of anxiety – many with a strong feeling that they are victims of a sexual situation which they are powerless to do anything about. Men often have dreams of bad luck and misfortune, but women tend to have dreams in which they're actually being put upon (usually by men). I must point out, however, that *all* dreams are preponderantly unhappy rather than happy (about 5:1), and so it's fruitless to expect joy and fun in every night's quota. What these anxious sexual dreams reflect is that women feel genuinely sexually repressed by men and don't quite know what they're going to do about it. In an astonishingly large number of sexual dreams, the woman feels herself to be a *victim*.

Mind you, I'm not saying that many women don't find it sexually exciting to be victimized. This is another ambivalent characteristic of woman's highly ambivalent psychological makeup. But it does show to what purpose most women's sexual dreams are directed, and what problem they are attempting to solve.

I dreamed my husband John was taking me to a party. It was being held in the house where I was brought up, in Cleveland, which surprised me. John insisted that I should take all my clothes off and go to the party naked, with a black hood over my head, and a silver chain around my neck which he would use to pull me along with. I begged and pleaded with him not to make me do it, but he didn't take any notice at all. I lay on the floor and kicked and shrieked, but he just looked out of the window.

The party itself seemed to begin all around us. It didn't seem like a very happy party. More like a wake. People were sitting all around looking very stiff and uncomfortable. They were drinking sherry out of very small glasses and mumbling under their breath. Everyone was dressed except me. I tried to keep still and quiet so that no one would notice me. But my wrists and ankles were chained, and every time I moved, they made a rattling noise which made everyone look around.

I knew most of the people there. My Aunt Roberta, my Uncle Peter, and the Greens from next door. My mother was around someplace as well, and I was terrified she was going to see me. John, my husband, seemed to have disappeared altogether, and I thought: 'What a rat, he's deserted me.'

A man I didn't know came over to talk to me. I knew he was aware of my nakedness, but he was trying to hide the fact that he knew. He reminded me of someone I knew very well, but for a long time I couldn't place him. Then I realized it was Clint Eastwood. We talked for awhile about new ways of potting plants. In the dream I seemed to know that he was an expert on potted plants, and that meant we shared an interest. But then he came up very close to me, and started unlacing the front of his pants. They were held together by a long kind of leather lace. I tried to push him away, but he had me wedged against the wall. He kept touching my nipples with the buckskin fringes on his sleeves, and that made my nipples tingle and pulse.

I looked down and he'd managed to work his prick out of his pants. It was very long and thin, just like him. It seemed to be shining as if it was covered in grease or oil. He looked around to make sure that everybody was busy someplace else, and then he forced his prick between my legs and into my cunt. I didn't want to be taken that way. I wanted to seduce him and do it properly. I told him I didn't want to be used as a piece of property, a piece of furniture to fuck whenever he felt like it, but he didn't take any notice.

He fucked me faster and faster, and the fringes on his sleeves brushed against my breasts and made them throb – like nettles or jellyfish tentacles. I lifted my legs right off the floor and wound them around his waist, and he was gripping the cheeks of my bottom and ramming his prick in and out of me as hard as he could. I knew I was going to have a climax, and that annoyed me, because I was going to have one in spite of myself – in spite of what I believed was the right way to do it.

I started shouting in Clint Eastwood's ear: 'I'm a person, you know! Women are people too!' But all he did was fuck me harder. Then I thought: 'My God – supposing I have Clint Eastwood's baby?'

When I felt him shoot his come inside, it felt so real that I didn't know if I was dreaming or not. You can never describe to a man what it's like when you feel sperm pouring out of your husband's prick, or your lover's – or your rapist's, I suppose. I woke up, and I was lying there covered in sweat, and my cunt was so juicy I hardly knew what to do. John said: 'What's the matter?' And I said: 'I just had a dream about Clint Eastwood.' And he said: 'Oh, that idiot,' and went back to sleep. But the dream was important to me. That's why I made a point of remembering it. It was the first dream that really told me I was underprivileged as a person. It was telling me that I saw myself as a fuck-object, and that's not exactly a pretty thing to be.

Many people still believe Freud's theory that dreams are provoked by unconscious wishes, and that what you experience in your dream is a wish-fulfillment. Our minds are crowded with sexual and aggressive lusts, he thought, which we normally repress during the day. But when we sleep, the barriers go down, and the deeply buried wishes rise closer to conscious thought. Some of the wishes, though, are so extreme that they appear in disguise — hidden by symbols and puns and metaphors. If they weren't disguised, claimed Freud, we would wake up in horror. Dreams are the guardian of our sleep. They wrap our wishes up in a candy coating that won't disturb us until our friendly neighborhood analyst comes along and tells us what nasty things are lurking beneath the sugar.

Of course, this wish-fulfillment theory (formulated in 1895) was a big step forward in psychology and in the investigation of dreams. But subsequent laboratory research has shown that it just isn't true. We dream in ninety-minute cycles, and it's highly unlikely that our unconscious mind is going to release a suppressed wish with such unvarying regularity. REM sleep has been shown to be a physiological process, rather than a psychological one, and is not in any way the result of suppressed wishes. As for dreams being the guardians of our sleep, we can only point to all those people who have slept quite happily through dreams of murder, incest, and rape and woke up feeling jolly and refreshed.

There are many different theories about why we dream, and what the contents of our dreams really mean. If you accept what Freud had to say — that dreams disguise unpleasant and horrifying desires with symbols and codes — then you're obviously going to believe that even the most ordinary dreams have deep significance. If, for instance, you dream of being prodded by a man carrying a rolled-up copy of *The Christian Science Monitor*, you're going to assume that this was a disguise for sexual assault. The dream may certainly have some sexual implications, but what you're really dreaming about is being prodded by a man with a rolled-up copy of *The Christian Science Monitor*.

Some researchers think that when we're dreaming, our

minds are like computers, programming and reprogramming the information that we've collected during the day. But if this were true — if we were really processing and filing in our sleep — then people who had less sleep, or interrupted sleep, would be less adapted to life and less psychologically integrated. We know that this isn't the case.

From all that we know about dreams up to date, they are nothing more than the fantasies of the mind as it mulls over the events and problems of the day. I say 'nothing more', but I don't mean that because dreams are not necessarily disguised lusts or coded wishes, they are unimportant. On the contrary, dreams bring a throng of unconscious ideas and responses to bear on the events of our waking life — ideas and responses that can tell us more about ourselves than almost any other form of human expression. As Freud said, dreams are the 'royal road to the unconscious.'

If the things and people that appear in your sexual dreams are not disguises and masks, then what are they? And why are your sexual dreams so peculiar? Why do you dream about having animals instead of babies or Clint Eastwood or your husband under the hood of a car?

Well, when you're asleep, your mind can range freely from conscious to unconscious levels, and there is no need for logic. All inspired and creative thoughts depend on our ability to think of thousands of different permutations, puns, analogies, and metaphors. Friedrich Kekule, the nineteenth-century German chemist, had a dream in which he visualized a snake eating its own tail — a dream which led him to discover that the six carbon atoms in a benzene molecule were arranged in a circle, rather than the straight line he had previously imagined. Astrologer Hugh Mac-Craig worked out a table in his sleep that would accurately predict the positions of the moon up until the year 2000.

If our brains weren't constantly comparing one idea with another, there wouldn't be any jokes, symbols, poetry, or progressive thought.

Because your dreams tend to revolve around the events of the day, and the problems that you're trying to work your way through at any particular moment, the images they contain are usually related to people and objects that are quite familiar to you. They may not appear exactly as they would in waking life, but if you think clearly about them, you won't find them hard to identify. Even Freud had to admit that plenty of dreams are quite plain, and don't need very much in the way of interpretation. All I'm warning you against is overinterpretation – trying to read significance into odd images and odd events that are really no more than puns or silly jokes. For instance, a 24-year-old New York girl dreamed that her uncle was walking down a corridor dressed in pink corsets. She immediately knew what the dream image was all about. Her uncle's favorite phrase was 'of *course* it is,' and when she was a little girl she had imagined he was saying 'of córset is.'

Now that it's been established that REM sleep cycles are a catalyst for dreams, and not the other way around, it's reasonable to assume that other natural cycles can affect the contents of your dreams. Your menstrual cycle, for example. Robert Van de Castle of the University of Virginia has undertaken studies which indicate that what you dream about is substantially conditioned by your time of the month. That's one factor that men have never had to take into consideration when they've been interpreting their dreams, but it's essential that women do. Later on, we'll see how you can include menstrual factors in your interpretation of sexual dreams.

I had a dream that I went to a very swank diplomatic ball. I was wearing a long evening dress in gorgeous blue silk, which left my breasts almost completely bare, and I was dripping with diamonds and sapphires. Everyone turned around to stare at me as I came in, and I really waggled my hips to show off. But halfway across the floor, I suddenly realized that they were staring because I had a red stain on the front of my dress. My period was starting!

I hid behind a group of people and went over to the buffet table. A man in a beautiful tuxedo was stirring a crystal bowl of punch with his cock. He brought it out of the punch, dripping with drink and with a round slice of orange peel hanging around the end. He said, 'It's delicious – would you care for some?' But I was too worried about my period. I stole as many napkins as I could, and started to stuff them up my dress. Then, across the other side of the room, I saw a beautiful naked man. I mean, he was really beautiful. Golden skin, curly hair, beautiful muscles. He was naked, and his cock was moving real graceful as he walked along. And there was I, crouched under the buffet table with my dress crammed with napkins.

Then I was home in Illinois. I don't know how I managed to get there. I could hear my father mowing the grass outside. I was locked in the bathroom, and the whole floor was covered in blood. I knew my mother was away in Chicago for the day, and I didn't know how I was possibly going to explain all this blood to my father. I started to cry, and I woke up with tears in my eyes.

Some dreams are affected by even more immediate stimuli. If you have pressure on your bladder, or if you're hungry or thirsty, or if your lover or husband has his arms around you as you sleep, or if there's a noise in the street outside, or if you can smell smoke or perfume, then you may find that related images filter their way into your dreams. 'I dreamed that I was having intercourse with my lover in the kitchen. The gas was on, and the heat was becoming intolerable. We were both sweating like you wouldn't believe. I woke up to find that the central heating was full on, and the thermostat was broken.'

Several women claim to have had sexual dreams which appeared to be precognitive or clairvoyante – in other words, the dreams appeared to predict the future or tell them something which they could not possibly have known. Dr Faraday quotes a woman who dreamed that she looked in the pocket of her husband's sports jacket and found a letter from another woman. When she woke up, she actually checked her husband's jacket, and sure enough – there was the letter.

Dreams like these seem to be caused by the unconscious mind letting us know things that, consciously, we would rather not know, or which we cannot consciously understand. When the girl who had had the 'letter dream' was questioned by her therapy group, it turned out that her husband had been away from home for several nights, he had stayed late at the office several times, and he had frequently put the phone down quickly when she came into the room. She admitted she may even have seen a letter in her husband's pocket and wondered what it was. Even though her conscious mind was not prepared to admit the suspicion of her husband's unfaithfulness, her unconscious mind certainly was. And that's why her dream occurred.

Similar mental processes occur with dreams that seem to foretell the future, as well as dreams that jog your memory about things which you thought you'd forgotten, and dreams that give you insights into the true nature of people you know. Here's an example from a 22-year-old Boston girl.

I dreamed about my lover, Bob. We were making love. It all seemed so real that I couldn't believe it was a dream, and yet somewhere in the back of my mind I knew that it was. We were lying on a strange bed somewhere – in a hotel, I think – and we were making love very lazily and pleasantly. I was lying on my back with my legs apart, and he was moving in and out of me with absolute grace. His body was rippling with every stroke, and I held on to the cheeks of his ass and I could feel him pushing into me.

I looked down at our bodies, and the whole idea of us two being together seemed perfect. The way his chest pressed against my breasts. The way his penis was sliding in and out of me. His pubic hair and his balls drawn up tight. Lovely. But then I looked up at his face, and he seemed to have hair all over it. I felt anxious and worried, and I looked some more, and then I understood what was going on. His head was kind of fixed on backwards, and what I was seeing was the back of his head.

He was talking to someone else. He was actually making love to me and talking to someone else at the same time. I suddenly thought to myself: 'What a fucking sham this man is. He's all style and nothing else.'

When I woke up, I wondered if I was being ridiculous. But the more I thought about this dream, the more it seemed to ring true. I'd been wondering for a long time if he really cared about me, but I'd never let myself admit it before. Now I knew what I really felt. There were so many little things that he'd done that I'd pretended not to notice, and all the time I'd been storing them up in the back of my mind. I broke our relationship off a few days later. I couldn't get that image of the back of his head out of my mind.

A typical 'reminder' dream comes from this 20-year-old New York girl:

I had a long and worrying kind of dream that seemed to go on for hours. Someone was talking in this dream, and trying to explain something to me. But I wasn't interested, or else I couldn't hear them properly. Then I was on my knees on the floor of my apartment, wearing a thin shirt and no other clothes at all. The windows were open, and outside it looked as though there was a storm brewing up. My shirt was flapping, and I was beginning to feel cold.

A man I used to know two or three years ago came into the room and walked up to me. He knelt down in front of me, and we had a whispered conversation that I couldn't quite hear. All the time, he kept leaning forward and kissing my neck and nuzzling around in my hair. I began to unbutton his shirt, and rub my hands across his chest. He was wearing tight jeans, and somehow I had translucent vision, and I could see his cock rising up inside them. I could see the dark red head of it, and I could

see the brown-colored shaft, and the black smudge of pubic hair.
It was like looking at them through mist.

He stood up, and he opened his pants by means of strange
triangular flaps. I thought to myself that this was a kind of
Japanese *origami*. He took out his cock, and it was just as
gorgeous and tasty as I always remembered. I closed my eyes and
opened my mouth for it, and he was just about to push it in
between my lips when I thought of something. I clapped my hand
over my mouth just in time to catch all my teeth as they crunched
and splintered into little pieces. I thought: 'I must phone the
dentist. I'll never to able to suck him off if I don't have my teeth
fixed.'

The next morning when I woke up, I remembered that I had a
dental appointment the day after. I'd forgotten all about it – and,
as usual, I'd forgotten to write it down. Somehow the dream,
right in the middle of a sexy scene, reminded me of what I had to
do.

Apart from the way in which this dream reminded the
girl of her dental appointment, I can't help being struck by
the possible dream pun *origami*. It has echoes of 'oral sex',
'orgy', and even the archaic word for fellatio, 'gamahuch-
ing', more commonly known these days as 'gamming'.

Sexual dreams about falling hair or dropping teeth are
not at all uncommon. They usually seem to represent a
sense of loss or failure, and it's possible that this girl's
dream had something to do with losing her one-time
boyfriend. After all, she seemed very pleased to see him
when he turned up.

As I remarked in the Prologue, there is no concrete
evidence that dreams can predict the future, and I'm
inclined to agree with Jung's opinion that they present us
with possibilities rather than firm predictions. Every decision we make in life is based on a quick mental computa-
tion of possible outcomes, so it's hardly surprising that we
should be doing the same thing in our dreams. Dreams
only seem to 'come true' when we happen to recall a
dream that closely resembled the incidents that have

actually occurred. We usually forget the dreams that predicted totally *different* possibilities. I'm not dismissing out of hand those people who claim to have had dreams about presidential assassinations, crashing airplanes, and earthquakes, but in a nation of 200 million people, it's odds-on that every night of the year someone, someplace, is dreaming about such things. One 27-year-old girl dreamed she was having intercourse with a Greek, and three days later she started dating a Turk, with whom she eventually went to bed. She liked to think that the dream was prophetic, but when she got down to analyzing it in more detail, she remembered that a friend of hers had asked her the day before she had the dream if she'd ever be prepared to gamble her life away 'like Nick the Greek.' The appearance of the amorous Turk was purely happenstance.

Prophetic sexual dreams are particularly associated with pregnancy and birth. Many women dream about conceiving and about having babies, and several joyful mothers have told me that they had a prophetic dream about the sex of their baby before it arrived. 'I *dreamed* it would be a boy,' they say, but when you consider they only have one other alternative, you can't in all fairness call their prophetic abilities a real wow. But, on the whole, pregnancy and birth dreams reveal fascinating aspects of any woman's character, whether she's maternally oriented or not, and they're worth paying very close attention to.

I dreamed I was sitting watching television. I was wearing jeans, but I was naked from the waist upwards. I had my hands on my stomach, and suddenly I felt something flutter inside it. I suddenly knew that I was going to have a baby. The only trouble was, I knew that it wasn't my husband's baby. It had come from a man I had met in California, when I went out there last year to visit a friend of mine. The man had been tall and blond, and he was nothing like my husband, so I knew that when the baby appeared, my husband would know straightaway that the baby wasn't his.

I decided to get rid of the baby. I went into the bathroom and took off my jeans, and I knelt down on the floor on all fours, propping a mirror up against the bath so that I could look between my legs and see my vagina. I started to make strange bubbling noises with my vagina, and then red and violet butterflies started to creep out from the lips of my vagina and fly around the bathroom. They were still sticky with vaginal juice, and they perched everywhere, quivering and waiting for their wings to dry. I knew there must be a baby inside me as well, so I pushed my hand carefully up my vagina until I felt something moving inside me. I got my hands around it, and tried to tug it out, but it seemed to resist. In the end, I had both hands up inside my vagina, and I was tugging and sobbing, and tugging and sobbing, and all the time I was terrified my husband was going to come home.

At last I managed to pull it right out of me. It wasn't a baby at all, but a huge hard penis, and a pair of very slippery testicles. I could only imagine that the man I had slept with in California had left them inside me when we made love, or else I had been giving birth to a boy, and the rest of his body had turned into butterflies, leaving just his penis and his testicles behind.

My husband came into the room. He stood there looking very pale. I tried to hide the penis behind my back, but he said, 'I know what you're holding there. You've been having babies again, haven't you?' I swore that I hadn't. But he led me through into the sitting room, and there, on the settee, all wrapped up in lace, was the man I had met in California, only he wasn't a man, he was just a tiny baby.

Much of this dream is explicit. The girl was obviously feeling residual guilt from her affair on the West Coast, and was also afraid that her husband might find out. The birth scene though, was very much more complicated in its implications, and it did not imply that she wanted a baby, either from her husband or her lover. Too many people assume that if a woman dreams about babies, she is a frustrated mother. Just as often, she is afraid of having children, afraid of her husband's desire to have children, or seeking some way of understanding her sexual identity as a woman. 'Being a woman and not having a baby is a very strange and anticlimactic thing,' a 34-year-old Hollywood actress told me. 'It's like bringing a gun into a movie and then never firing it.' But do you *have* to have a baby just because you *can*? No wonder it's a topic for sexual dreams.

After pregnancy and conception, lesbianism is another dream topic that alarms many women. Just because they dream about kissing other women or having sexual liaisons with them, they believe that they're turning 'queer'. But just like birth dreams, lesbian dreams are only another way of locating your female identity — and if it's any consolation, men have just as many dreams of sex with other men.

I was driving through France in a wonderful open-topped touring car. It had a long sleek hood, and it was a glittering red. The year was 1931. I was sure of that, although I don't know how I was sure of it. There were three other girls in the car with me, and we were all beautifully dressed in 1930s clothes. Long white scarves, cloche hats, loose cotton dresses in pale greens and whites and rusts.

The road was straight and long, with rows of tall poplar trees on either side, and you could see as far ahead of you as you could behind. The sun was low, and the shadows from the poplar trees made stripes across the road. I could even smell the grass and the flowers, and see the cows stirring in the fields. It was so vivid that when I think about it I'm almost sad that it was only a dream, and that I was never really there. How can you dream about something so vividly when you've never actually been there? I wasn't even *alive* in 1931.

I'm talking to the other girls in French. Then the scene changes and we're sitting by the banks of the Loire. The river is drifting by, and I can hear bells tolling in the distance. We've opened a picnic hamper, and there's red wine and cold pheasant and cakes and pies. One of the girls sitting opposite me reminds me of a girl I used to go to school with. She was always very pretty, and her name was Suzanne. She was sitting with her legs raised, and I looked across and I could see her cunt. She wasn't wearing any panties. I was fascinated, and even though I knew that she knew I was looking, I couldn't take my eyes away from her. I could see everything, her furry pubic hair, her clitoris, and her pink lips which were slightly open. She was sitting on the grass, and the blades of grass were touching and tickling her cunt, and somehow the thought of that made me very sexually excited.

I went over to where Suzanne was sitting, and I raised my glass of wine. Then I pulled up her dress and poured it all over her cunt. She parted her legs and lifted her cunt towards the wine, and rolled her eyes with pleasure. 'You've spilled your wine,' she said. 'You ought to lick it off.' The other two girls, both of them laughing, came over and held up Suzanne's dress for me. They were pretty, too, with lovely eyes and long chestnut curls.

Suzanne raised her hips up as far as she could, and opened the sides of her cunt with her fingers, stretching it apart so that I could dip my tongue in. I felt hot and flushed, but I knew that I wanted to do it. I held my necklace in one hand to stop it swinging, then I knelt down and buried my head between her legs. To my surprise, her cunt kissed me back. It was like a mouth. We kissed each other for a long time, cunt to mouth, and I licked her and nipped her with my teeth. I was very aware of the fact that now I knew what a girl's cunt actually tasted like. It was a little like lobster. You expect it to be fishy, but it isn't at all. It's sweet and watery and cold. That's what Suzanne's cunt tasted like.

I turned around and the other two girls had lifted up my dress, and they were sticking their fingers in my cunt and my asshole, and giggling as if they were eight years old. I was sure that I wasn't supposed to be doing things like this, but I was enjoying myself. I was having great surges of sexual pleasure, and I began to wonder if I was going to have an orgasm. All of a sudden, the sky grew very dark and it began to rain. We were soaked in just a few seconds, and I knew that I had to put the tonneau cover on the car, or the seats would be ruined. I took the hamper and went over to where I thought the car was, and my husband was standing there, looking very angry, with a basketful of cucumbers.

This, the lesbian dream of a 25-year-old New York wife, is a very pretty dream, and even though there is some anxiety towards the end, it has a romantic and idyllic quality which sexual dreams don't often have. This is particularly interesting when you consider that the girl is not an overt or practising lesbian in waking life, and has been quite happily married for two years. It's possible that the masculine side of her sexual character is emerging in her dream – a masculine side that would certainly think of a ride in the country with three beautiful girls as a treat. I like the phallic basket of cucumbers, which the irate husband seems to be carrying as a very obvious reminder that he is the one with the penis.

Jung postulated that women have a masculine element in their makeup, their *animus*, while men have a feminine element, their *anima*. The animus is the logical, deductive, and intellectual aspect of a woman's personality which our culture teaches her to neglect. To become a whole personality, she must use her contacts with men to cultivate her animus, and it will help her to develop self-knowledge, judgement, and the ability to reflect and deliberate. The anima, which the man must develop through his contacts with women, is the source of emotion, instinctive reaction, warmth, and intuition. To my mind, dreams of homosexuality and lesbianism are often an expression of the masculine or feminine characteristics within your personality – characteristics which, when you're asleep, are not rigidly repressed by social convention and morality, as they are when you're awake. They don't necessarily signify that you're a lesbian. They simply reveal within your own personality the male personality, which is capable of appreciating other women sexually as well as platonically.

So far, we have touched only on the mainstream contents of women's sexual dreams, and we have not attempted to interpret them in any detail. What I have principally tried to show you is that women's erotic dreams, if they are going to be explored with any depth, must be seen as separate creations from the dreams of men. The objects and the people that women dream about, the way they dream about them, and even the times when they dream about them are often substantially different.

We have seen what women dream about most when they are having sex dreams — the kinds of problems that usually occupy their unconscious thoughts. A lot of the time it's marriage and security and birth and pregnancy — the kind of cozy sexual situations that most men would assume that you dream about. But you don't usually dream about them in a cozy way, and you also dream about such prickly erotic topics as incest and lesbianism and finding your sexual freedom.

It's possible to analyze what women dream about down to the last symbol and image, and Professor Calvin S. Hall has prepared several lists of people, animals, events, and objects that have appeared in his subjects' dreams. I notice that Chester (from *Gunsmoke*) turns up in one woman's dreams, along with opossums, caterpillars, barnacles, and hamsters. When you're dealing with your own sexual dreams, however, it's more reliable to compile your own personal lists and not try to relate the contents of your dreams to anyone else's.

You see, despite the fact that you have a limited number of main types of sex dream, the actions you perform in individual dreams are many and varied, and extremely idiosyncratic. 'Two of the most interesting features of sex dreams are the great variety of sexual activity that takes place and the great diversity of partners with whom the dreamer has sexual interactions. One dreamer had sexual intercourse with a knothole, one experienced orgasm while climbing a tree, a third ejaculated while he was walking along a railroad track. Dreamers engage in coitus, anal intercourse, fellatio, cunnilingus, analingus, and others.

Foreplay includes kissing, embracing, caressing the breasts, and so forth.'

That's how Professor Hall reports the sexual dreams of some of his male subjects. Now let's see just how rich and varied the sexual dreams of women can be.

2

Ten Common Erotic Dreams

Before you start to analyze your erotic dreams in any detail, it's essential that you try to understand what kind of a dream it is. The interpretation of many of the images and events that occur in your dreams can differ, according to whether they're dreams of rape, marriage, incest, or whatever. As a simple example, you wouldn't interpret the appearance of a policeman in a rape dream in the same way that you would interpret his appearance in a marriage dream. He would probably represent official authority in both dreams but in completely different ways. The same goes for any dream character or object – whether it's your father and mother, a cucumber, or a railroad tunnel.

Usually, it's fairly easy to decide what kind of a sexual dream you've just had, especially if the emotions involved have been very strong. 'I dreamed I was married to James Caan,' said a Cleveland housewife. 'When I woke up, I couldn't believe that I was still me and not the new Mrs Caan.'

But sometimes, there are several different themes running through the same dream. Or else the theme may change in mid-dream, and what started out as a cozy dream of marriage turns into a scarifying dream of sexual assault. In these events, you will have to choose the strongest theme, and try to interpret your dream along those lines. If your interpretation doesn't seem to ring true when you've done that, then pick out a subordinate theme and see how that fits.

You're obviously beginning to appreciate that you are the most important guide and analyst when it comes to solving the meaning of your erotic dreams. There are several reasons for this. First, you are the only person who has ever experienced the dream at firsthand, with all its sounds and sights and smells and associations. Second, the dream comes entirely from within your mind, and only you have the ability to decide whether a dream situation really reminds you of something in your waking life or not. Your psychoanalyst, as far as your erotic dreams are concerned, can never be anything more than a commentator. He is in the same position as a doctor trying to tell a ship's captain how to take the first mate's appendix out over ship-to-shore radio. He obviously has expert knowledge and experience that may be able to help you make your interpretation. After all, many women have similar dreams and he's probably come across most types of dreams before. But the final interpretation must always be yours. Only you can tell whether it feels right or not. When Dr Ann Faraday was undergoing training analysis from a Freudian doctor, he interpreted her love of her career as a need for a substitute penis and suggested that her true fulfillment lay in becoming 'a real woman' and devoting her life to looking after her husband and her family. She became so brainwashed by this suggestion that when her husband demanded she make a choice between home and career, she gave up her work and tried to be the perfect housewife. The result of that was frustration and depression, and it was only when her marriage broke up and she resumed her work that she found happiness and satisfaction again.

'My analyst had insisted on doing a job I had not asked him to do by treating my career as a symptom. He used his Freudian theories like a hammer, trying to refurnish my life with his own (and Freud's) theories about what a "real woman" should be.'

She persisted with Freudian analysis with another

doctor, but she was eventually made ill 'by the analyst's constant Procrustean efforts to make me fit a theory in which women are expected to sacrifice their individuality and initiative to the service of men.'

As Eva Figes said in *Patriarchal Attitudes*: 'The "cured" patient is actually brainwashed, a walking automaton, as good as dead. The corners have been knocked off and the woman accepts her own castration, acknowledges herself as inferior, ceases to envy the penis and accepts the passive role of femininity. Sadly, man recognizes that the ideal, submissive woman he has created for himself is somehow not quite what he wanted. Freud's basic view was that every woman was a square peg trying to fit a round hole. It did not occur to him that it might be less destructive to change the shape of the holes rather than to knock all the corners off.'

I'm sure you're not going to let yourself wind up as a walking automaton, but when it comes to deciding what your erotic dreams mean, just remember that you are your own best analyst.

One of the most important things to remember when you're interpreting your erotic dreams is that, with dreams, there are no easy answers. It's tricky enough trying to decide what general classification your dream might belong to, let alone putting precise meanings on images and symbols that occurred within the dream. Because your unconscious mind is working on many different levels of awareness at once, then it's probable that most dreams have a multiplicity of different meanings. Anyone who says that they know exactly what your sexual dreams are all about is talking rubbish, and so by the same token are those 'dream dictionaries' that dogmatically tell you that to dream of seeing a mustache shaved off means an unhappy sexual experience ahead. I'm not dismissing dream dictionaries out of hand, because their interpretations are often based on quite sensible classic analyses that go back thousands of years. But I do suggest that you measure their interpretation up against yours, and if you prefer yours, to gently discard what they say.

Never force an interpretation or a classification on a dream that you can't quite fathom. Later on, we'll see how you can assemble an erotic dream diary with your dreams entered in series, and you will frequently find that when you see a dream in context with other dreams you've had, its meaning becomes much clearer. Let's face it, the events of a single day of waking existence, when studied in isolation, would seem just as eccentric and meaningless as a dream. Why did you buy so many steaks at an unfamiliar supermarket? Why did you telephone that strange man in Hyannis? Why did that girl put her head around your apartment door and say, 'They're coming up'? Unless you knew that you had friends coming to dinner, and you had to do your marketing in a different neighborhood because your job took you out of town that day, and you had to call a tax consultant in Massachusetts to confirm the deal you were making, and when you got home your roommate wanted to tell you your friends would be coming up soon, those incidents would seem peculiar and quite irrational. Each dream you can remember is only a fragment of a much longer mental experience, and you must think of it as a clue, rather than a whole story. Like a detective, the more clues you assemble, the more chance you have of solving the mystery.

I dreamed I was lying in a huge double bed in a strange house. The early morning sunlight was just coming through the curtains, and there was a sound like birds singing outside. I turned over and I wasn't sure if I was asleep or awake — whether I'd really woken up and I was actually here, in this strange bed, or whether I was still asleep. It was so vivid. I could even feel the crispness of the pillow against my cheek.

Lying next to me, fast asleep, was a rather handsome young man. He had dark curly hair, and he looked as if he was Italian or something like that. He was naked, and I started caressing the black hairs on his chest, and feeling down his thighs and between his legs. His penis was soft at first, but then it started to grow in the palm of my hand, and it grew bigger and bigger until it raised the blankets off the bed. All the time, the man was still asleep, although I wondered if he was really pretending.

Then I heard whispering, and I realized it was coming from an old Cathedral radio on the dresser. Somehow I was standing next to it, trying to hear what it was saying. I was naked, too, although I tried to hide my breasts with two blue-and-yellow drinking mugs. I knew the radio was saying something about *sex and spaghetti, sex and spaghetti*, and *don't forget the tomatoes, Doreen*. Then I woke up.

This, the dream of a 27-year-old secretary from St Augustine, Florida, completely foxed her at first. It was only when she had a second and third dream about different aspects of the same incident that the meaning began to penetrate through.

In one of the dreams, I thought I was sitting in the small garden of my brother's house in Orlando. It was a very hot day, and I was wearing a white flouncy dress. I knew my brother was inside the house someplace, but I didn't want to go inside, in case he was kissing his bride. Well, I'd call her his *wife* these days, but in the dream it seemed to me that he'd only just gotten married. Her name's Florence, and she's very pretty and sexy.

But somehow I couldn't resist walking in. There didn't seem to be anyone around. Then I looked over the edge of the settee, and there was Florence naked, with her legs wide apart, and my brother on top of her, making love to her. I stood there, feeling embarrassed and fascinated, and I couldn't take my eyes off them. I'd never seen anyone making love before, and it turned me on. I knelt down on the floor, lifted up all my flounces, and frantically started to diddle myself.

In another dream, I was walking through a strange neighborhood. I didn't know where I was, and I was worried in case I got home late. My brother was standing on a street-corner, waiting for me. I knew that something was wrong. He took out his penis and laid it in my hand. His penis started to pour out dollops of white come, which filled up the palm of my hand and dripped to the sidewalk.

There are countless different ways of interpreting these dreams. If you interpret them individually, like dream dictionaries tend to do, you can come up with some pretty odd answers. Dreams of spaghetti, says one book, are a forecast of gay social times, especially if you drip the sauce on yourself. Tomatoes are a sign of happiness and contentment. A quiet radio foretells family harmony. Another dream book says that two cups indicate the Terrible Mother, one of Jung's archetypal dream characters, and this dictionary interpretation came reasonably close to the truth. The Terrible Mother is entwining, devouring, and possessive – a mother who keeps her children incestuously bound to her.

This girl's dreams did have their incestuous side. They were dreams of sexual jealousy about her brother, with whom she had always been very close. The first dream, in a strange house, was an idealized dream of what it would have been like if she had married her brother herself. But she doesn't recognize him as her brother because he has become Italian. He has married Florence. Only the girl herself could know that the name 'Florence' always reminded her of a schoolbook picture of Italy, with crowds of Italians in the foreground. The old radio was the radio she and her brother had listened to in their childhood, and the blue-and-yellow drinking mugs, which she had consciously forgotten, were a pair of mugs that she and her brother had been given when they were very small. It was only when the girl mentioned the mugs to her mother that their relevance became clear.

The two succeeding dreams make the incest theme clearer. The third dream relates to the first quite closely.

The girl was sent out to buy groceries in a strange neighborhood when she was eight years old. She got lost and her brother was sent out to find her. She dropped a bagful of eggs, and her brother had poured the contents of one egg into the palm of her hand.

There are more details in the dream, and they yielded more and more information as the girl thought further about the implications of her incestuous love. But they need not concern us right now. The point is clear enough. The more dreams you manage to remember, the clearer their meaning will become. And there is only one person who can make the leaps of imagination and association necessary to solve the riddle of your sexual dreams, and that is you.

We can use these dreams to explain how to classify your sexual dreams, too. It's clear that the overriding theme was incest, and therefore, all the images and the events could be understood in relation to that theme. The radio, the blue-and-yellow mugs, and so on. But there is also an element of voyeurism in the dream (catching her brother and his bride *in flagrante delicto*) and masturbation, as well as a faint but discernible trace of masochistic or at least submissive behavior (the come in the palm of the hand).

From all the erotic dreams that I have gathered together, the predominating themes are those which I mentioned in the previous chapter – rape, marriage, birth, nudity, celebrities, incest, orgasm, sadomasochism, lesbianism, and sexual freedom. This doesn't mean that women have erotic dreams only about these themes, but I think you will find that the bulk of your nocturnal fantasies fit someplace into these patterns.

To give you some idea of how to put your dream into a rough classification, here are ten dreams that women have reported, one in each of the ten classifications. You will be able to pick out underlying themes of other sexual predilections, but you will soon be able to see why they were classified in the way they were. Remember that this classification is the first important step in accurate dream interpretation, and until you have acquired the talent of slotting your dreams into the right pigeonhole, understanding them in detail will always be more of a problem.

First, here is a classic rape dream, from a 23-year-old sculpture student from Berkeley, California:

In my dream, I was trying to finish a clay model, and for some reason the clay kept sticking to my tools and making it impossible for me to work with it. I was growing more and more frustrated, and in the end I decided I would have to leave. The sculpture room was empty, and everyone else seemed to have gone home. I went to the door and tried to open it, but it was locked in a peculiar way, and there was nothing I could do to budge it. I began to grow anxious, and wonder if there was anybody around who could let me out.

I think I managed to climb out of a window. I'm not quite sure now. But then I was crossing the open ground between the college buildings. I knew that I wasn't supposed to be there at that time of night, and I tried to hurry as fast as I could, but my legs seemed to be glued to the ground. It was cold, and the clouds were going very fast up above me.

Then I knew that someone was chasing me. I felt really frightened, and my heart almost seized up. I tried to run away, but the more effort I made to escape, the more gluey the ground seemed to get. It wasn't long before I could hear footsteps and heavy breathing behind me, and I knew that some men called Biloxi were after me. Don't ask me why they were called Biloxi, or how I knew, but that was their name, and it frightened me.

I thought I might be able to run between a row of hedges and get away. I seemed to get very light, and I floated along, but it was difficult to go very fast because my toes only touched the ground now and again. Suddenly one of the Biloxi men caught me, and the grass seemed to open up into a dark envelope and we plunged into it. It's hard to describe it, the way it actually was.

We were all standing in an elevator. Me in the middle, and all these men, these huge hairy men, pressing in on me from all sides. I could even smell them. They were big and hard and very powerful, and although I can't remember what their faces were like, I know that they were staring at me and licking their lips.

Between them, three or four of the men lifted me up. I could actually feel their hands gripping my arms and legs. I struggled, but they seized my panties and pulled them down, and then they tore off my bra and what was left of my dress. I know I was begging and whimpering. I have never begged or whimpered like that in my whole life, and somehow it almost turned me on, the thought that I was completely at the mercy of these men, nude and frightened, and that they could do anything they wanted with me. So all I could do was beg and pray. It seemed even sexier that begging and praying didn't have any effect.

One of the men grabbed hold of my waist and lifted me up again, until I was holding on to the shoulders of another man. Then another man produced this massive prick. It was so huge that it was almost a joke. There's a drawing by Aubrey Beardsley called *The Lacedemonian Ambassadors*, and they all have pricks like that.

The men all started grunting, and some of them were openly beating their meat. The man who was holding me up started moving me around until he had my cunt positioned over the prick of this man who was going to rape me. I knew, in the dream, that I was going to get hurt. I wanted to be hurt, in a way, yet on the other hand I was terrified of it. These men all smelled like goats, and their hair was wiry like the inside of an old mattress.

One man was now standing in front of me, holding me right up in the air by gripping my legs under the knees and raising his arms. That meant that I was hanging in mid-air with my legs up and my cunt stretched wide apart, and there was nothing I could do about it. The man who was holding me started to drop me down towards the prick of the man who was going to rape me. I looked down between my legs and I could actually see this huge purple prick trying to force its way inside me. It was like giving birth in reverse. The thing pushed and pushed until it finally started to sink inside me, and I just watched as I sank lower and lower down on it, right down to the man's pubic hair, which was as rough as a doormat.

The sexual feeling was extraordinary. I had a terrible fear that my hole was never going to be the same again. But at the same time, I almost thought it was worth it. It was so erotic. I mean, such a turn-on. I clung on to this Biloxi man's enormous prick, and I tried to touch the ground with my toes, but his prick was so solidly up inside me, and he was so tall, that I couldn't quite make it.

But I knew I couldn't stay there much longer. I was feeling precarious and I was starting to fall. If only he would come to a climax and let me down. He started kissing me, and to my horror, his mouth was a hairy asshole. He kept pressing it against my mouth, and it was all wrinkled and it tasted bitter, like shit. Then he came, deep inside me, and it was like hot water bubbling out of a faucet. I don't remember much more, and I think I woke up soon after. My bed was soaked with sweat, and my hand was deep down between my legs. I couldn't tell you for sure, but it almost seemed as though I'd been masturbating in my sleep.

This dream contains several very common rape-dream images. The feeling of being alone, in some place that's out of bounds; the feeling of being pursued and being unable to get away; the feeling of helplessness; and the feeling of being a sexual victim. The feeling of disgust and pain and irrevocable physical damage, coupled with intense sexual excitement and real erotic arousal.

I think it's worth pointing out that rape dreams and fantasies should not be confused with how a woman really feels about the prospect of rape. Many women and girls dream about rape, some have erotic daydreams about it, but that doesn't mean for a moment that they have any taste for the real thing. Most of these fantasies feature men that the girl already knows and likes, or movie stars she thinks are attractive and sympathetic. Or even if they don't, and the men are totally brutal and uncompromising, there is still enough sexual arousal in the dreams or fantasies to make them exciting and acceptable. Rape, in real life, is not acceptable, and I don't want you to think that I'm excusing it on the grounds that you sometimes have turn-on dreams about it.

While we're still examining this particular dream, let's note some of the other sexual themes in it apart from rape. There's a hint of bestiality (the smelly, goat-like men), and there's also a hint of birth (the enormous penis). The final sequence, when the rapist's mouth turns out to be an anus, could be interpreted as submission (ass kissing), but I wouldn't like to put too glib an interpretation on it until the girl explains her own associations. She might have kissed a boyfriend in this way and been secretly repelled by what she had done — a feeling she had managed to suppress until it floated out in her dream.

The frustration of the sculpture that wouldn't turn out right and the locked door were both symptomatic of sexual and career problems. She was beginning to doubt her ability as an artist, and she was also worried that she was making a mess of her life. If she wasted time sculpting, the dream was telling her, she might find the door to other opportunities was locked. At least, that's one interpretation. The main point is that the basic theme of the dream was rape, and it can now be classified as a rape dream.

Now let's take a look at a marriage-and-home dream. We've already remarked that these dreams are not the cozy, fireside fantasies of would-be housewives. Women are often better at facing up to the realities of marriage than men, and when we plunge into their unconscious (and therefore uncensored) thoughts, we come right up against the nitty-gritty.

Here's the marriage-and-home dream of a 25-year-old housewife from Bangor, Maine:

I dreamed I was sitting at home with my husband Tom. I had the feeling that it was snowing outside. Tom had no clothes on, and he was playing with himself, and looking at his penis in a small hand-mirror. I kept trying to talk to him, and interest him in what I'd been doing during the day, because I knew there was something very important which I had to tell him. But he wouldn't listen — he went on playing with his penis and his balls and watching himself in the mirror.

I thought that if I exposed myself to him I could attract his attention. I lifted up my dress, and I remember that I pulled my panties to one side, and showed him my vagina. He still wouldn't look at me, and I kept trying to shout out to him. I even whistled. But he wouldn't pay me any attention at all.

I went upstairs and into our bedroom to look for something. I don't know what it was now, but I know that it was very important at the time. It was something to do with sex. The bedroom seemed to be damp and cold, and there was a kind of clinging fog in the air. The bedspread was stiff and frozen, like when you hang it out to dry on a frosty night.

I looked out of the upstairs window, and I saw Tom in the outhouse. He was still naked, and he seemed to have someone with him. He was talking for a long time, but I couldn't hear a word he was saying. Then I saw a dark-haired girl, with very big breasts and a curvy figure, and she was putting her arms around him and kissing him. I thought to myself 'That's the Girl in My Dreams.'

I found myself in the kitchen next, and I was opening all the doors of all the cupboards. The chinaware was as frail as powder and crumbled away to dust when I touched it. Then the kitchen door opened and Tom came in. He was still naked, and his penis was standing up. I knew that he couldn't have had sex with the Girl in My Dreams because he would have lost his erection.

I sat on the rim of the sink, and he cut my panties apart with scissors. Then he stood between my legs and pushed his penis up into my vagina. He felt like he always used to — warm and hard and lovely. He pushed in and out of me, gorgeous sexy long strokes, and I could feel the bumpy head of his penis going in and out. He whispered beautiful words to me, like how much he loved and needed me, and I closed my eyes and just felt that penis going in and out, and I pressed my hips as near to him as I could.

Just as he was coming, I looked across the kitchen and saw myself in the mirror. I had a weird creepy feeling, because in the mirror I looked just like the girl with the dark hair and the big breasts. In fact, I *was* her. I was someone different. Tom wanted me because I was some other girl. I looked across to the door, and the real me was walking in, and staring at both of us in real surprise and disgust. I didn't know which was me and which wasn't. We were just starting to argue about it, and open cans of sardines at the same time, when I woke up. My last thought was: We can't waste time while we're arguing, we must do something useful at the same time.

Although this dream has some puzzling symbols and images in it, it is fundamentally a straightforward portrait of a marriage under stress. The principal points aren't hard to decipher. The husband whose sex life has become selfish and remote. The marriage bed that has become cold and unpleasant. The wife's desperate attempts to attract her husband's attention again. The chinaware, a symbol of domesticity and married peace, collapsed into dust.

What was interesting about this dream was that the wife was not consciously aware of any sexual stress in the marriage. She may have unconsciously recognized the fatal signs, but her conscious mind was keeping a pretty firm lid on her fears. This is a good example of a warning dream – a dream that presents you with the facts as you know them, but as you are not prepared, in your waking life, to accept them.

The wife thought at first that the dark-haired 'Girl in My Dreams' was mystical evidence of another woman in her husband's life. But the scene in the kitchen gives a clearer indication of who she really is. She is in fact the wife herself *as she would like to be*. She is the sort of girl she thinks her husband would be attracted to. If only she could be like that, she would be able to turn him on and rekindle his dying sexual interest in her.

Opening the cans of sardines? Well, who knows? Not every event in every dream is full of weighty significance. She might simply have been responding to the kitchen situation by doing something practical. It's possible that this event was a neat way of underlining the fact that she had discovered her husband was a cold fish, but it's not worth laboring a dream image if you're already in possession of the most important aspects of the dream.

To my mind, marriage-and-home dreams are among the most useful and important of women's sexual dreams, and they should never be taken lightly. If you value your home situation, and you value your relationship with the man you love, then take heed. Your dreaming mind might be trying to tell you something very urgent and significant.

Celebrity dreams are among my favorite sexual dreams. It is always amusing to come across some well-known actor or entertainer or politician, actually playing a part in the erotic fantasies they have themselves helped to create. Celebrity dreams, surprisingly, don't always feature a woman's favorite celebrities, which leads me to think that the celebrity may be there to make a point about an everyday problem in the mind, rather than to fulfill a subconscious wish to meet him and make love to him. In other words, they've been roped in by Nocturnal Central Casting because they happen to fit the drama that your sleeping mind wants to play out.

I particularly like the wonderful informality which exists between dreamers and the celebrities they dream about. One of the more fascinating books about dreams, *Dreams About H. M. The Queen*, illustrates this perfectly. Ordinary British housewives seem to dream about little else except having their monarch around for cups of tea and currant buns and chatting about the latest local scandals.

Popular male actors figure fairly largely in women's sexual celebrity dreams. Telly Savalas, Robert Redford, Steve McQueen, Paul Newman, James Caan, Marlon Brando. But I liked the dream that follows, from a 30-year-old shoestore assistant in New York, because it had the flavor of something a little different:

I was working at the store and we were very busy. Then I realized that the guy I was serving was President Ford. He was sitting there in a shiny gray suit, with a carnation in his buttonhole, and he had one shoe off and one shoe on, and he was waiting for a fitting.

I said, 'Oh, hello, sir, what kind of shoe were you looking for?' and he said, 'A whore's brogue, please.' I understood what he meant in the dream, although I'm damned if I can understand it now. I said, 'Certainly, sir.' I sat down on the little seat, and I took his foot in my hand, and I measured his foot for size. It was pretty complicated and difficult, because I had a new kind of foot measurer, but in the end I managed to work out that his foot measured 1976. I said, 'That's very good, your foot measures the same as the bicentennial year,' and he said, 'Of course – why do you think they made me President?' And do you know, I really thought that was the answer. I thought I'd actually discovered why it was they made him President.

I was holding his foot in my hand, but he started to wriggle it. I looked at him to see what he was playing at, but he was just sitting there with his arms crossed and smiling at me. I smiled back, but his foot kept on wriggling around, and I couldn't manage to fit a shoe on it for love nor money.

President Ford leaned forward and he whispered, 'Tug your skirt down.' I said, 'What?' and he said, 'Tug your skirt down.' So I tugged my skirt down, and he wriggled that foot of his right up it, and his toes started tickling me between the legs. It was a real sexy feeling, and I tried to ask him to stop, but somehow the words wouldn't come. I thought, 'Well, he's the President, and I guess I ought to let him do it if he wants.' Somehow he managed to work his big toe into my panties, and he forced it into my snatch. His toe seemed as big as a cock, and I was getting so excited that I was feeling faint. He had his big toe right up in my snatch, and the rest of his toes were wriggling up and down on my clit, and I kept on looking around to make sure nobody was watching us.

Round about then, President Ford took hold of me and pulled my face down into his lap. His pants were open and his cock was sticking out of them, and he pushed my face right down on it, so all I could do was open my mouth and take his cock right in there. He was talking to me all the time. He was saying, 'You know, it's a great honor to be sucking a President's cock.' And I was trying to answer him, and tell him that I always voted Democrat, but he wouldn't let me up.

I was saved for a while by a herd of elk which had strayed into the store. I knew they were the President's personal responsibility, so I pointed them out to him. He lifted me on to the back of one of the elks, and then climbed up after me. He made sure he pushed his cock in between the cheeks of my ass, so that he'd get his rocks off as we rode along. You can't say he wasn't an opportunist.

We rode through some forests and then across a wide timber bridge. In the end we reached a kind of suburb, and we turned into the drive of a small white-painted house. The elk wasn't an elk any more, it had somehow turned itself into a car. President Ford said, 'This is the White House.' I was disappointed. I said, 'It's just an ordinary house,' and he said, 'What did you expect, a palace?'

We went inside and somehow it turned into my own house. We walked through to the bedroom. I was worried because I was taking the President home with me, and I didn't have any cookies or cake left. I noticed the floor of the bedroom was strewn with strange-colored fluff, all kinds of shapes and sizes. President Ford said, 'Well – are we going to go to bed?'

He looked pretty good when he was naked. I was surprised how young and smooth his body was. I said, 'You may be the President of these United States, but I set the pace in bed, and that's all there is to it.' I stood on the bed, and unbuttoned my dress down the front. I tossed it across the room. President Ford clapped and smiled, just like he does on the television. I was surprised that he was so like he was on the television. Then I took off my bra, and I flung that across the room. All the time I was humming the music from *The Stripper*. Dah-dah-dah, dum-dah dum-dah . . .

President Ford was licking his lips. I knew he wanted me. I held my breasts in my hands and I bounced them in front of his face. I have big breasts. They're kind of soft, but they're still big. Then I put my thumbs in my panties and started to edge them down, real slow and tempting, and President Ford had his eyes wide open and he was gripping his own cock so tight that it was almost black at the end.

I lay back on the bed and I kicked my legs in the air, so that he could see my snatch. He climbed on top of me and he started to fuck me, but apart from a faint kind of pleasant feeling, I couldn't feel his cock at all. I said, 'I can't feel your cock. Did you put it in me?' He looked kind of embarrassed and said, 'That's the problem. I have an invisible cock. I borrowed it from David McCallum, and he borrowed mine.'

I guess I should've thought this was funny, but in the dream it seemed very sad and serious. I lay there and I started to cry. President Ford was stroking my hair, and whispering nice things to me, but it didn't help. Then the telephone rang, and even before I answered it, someone said, 'It's not invisible, it's divisible.' And that was all. I woke up.

I hardly have to tell you that this dream was nothing to do with the real President Ford, and that it shouldn't in any way be taken as a reflection on his personal or executive conduct. The 'President Ford' of the dream is simply an image supplied by this woman's unconscious to fit the part of a confident and powerful man. It could just as easily have been Nelson Rockefeller or Teddy Kennedy or Tarzan.

This long dream is crammed with fascinating images, several of which bear much closer scrutiny. More than one dream dictionary rates the elk as a symbol of sexuality, and that's one interpretation that they may have got right in this case. Then there's the strange invisible penis. Invisibility in dreams is a sign of mysticism and spiritual power. And there's the strange-colored fluff, and the toe-job in the shoe store, not to mention the oddly stilted jokes – like thinking of voting Democrat while she's fellating a Republican president, and the idea of borrowing an invisible penis from David (*The Invisible Man*) McCallum.

Whatever these images add up to, the main theme of the dream is a sexual encounter with a celebrity. A celebrity who represents power and establishment. When the woman delved further into her own motivation for dreaming the dream, she was fairly sure that it had something to do with her desire for a man who would really look after her. (She was divorced from her first husband, who had been a pretty weak-willed type.) It wasn't a wish-fulfillment dream, however. It was a dream that postulated a particular situation, and gave her the chance to think how she might feel about it. It was one of a series of dreams, all superficially unconnected, but all basically linked to her anxiety about the future, her sexual frustration and her lonesomeness.

If you dream about a celebrity, you may be doing nothing more than whimsically casting a famous and attractive person in the leading role of your nocturnal theater. But you may also be considering what it would be like if a particular kind of sexual personality or situation entered your life. It might be Raquel Welch or Sophia Loren, it might be John Wayne or Dustin Hoffman. It might even be Woody Allen. But whoever it is, you're not really dreaming about sexual relations with him personally – only with the kind of person that they usually represent.

Now let's take a look at a birth-and-pregnancy dream. Birth-and-pregnancy dreams aren't always erotic in the sense of being exciting and arousing, but they almost always contain an underlying element of sexual satisfaction. They're often strongly exhibitionistic, too. Some women have very vivid dreams of gynecological examinations, and other dream of proudly producing a baby and saying: 'There – look what I've done!'

It isn't really surprising that the idea of conceiving and giving birth has its erotic side. The compulsion to reproduce is still strong within us, and not many women realize that their husbands are actually turned on by the thought of giving them a baby, and quite commonly by the sight of their pregnant stomachs.

Men sometimes dream of being pregnant themselves. I was given a very convincing account of gestation and parturition by a 54-year-old farmer from Nebraska. But a woman's dream of pregnancy and birth has a particular meaning and insight all of its own, and there is a sexual identity to it that a man's dream can never hope to have. It's the same when women dream of having a penis – they never get inside that odd and special relationship that men have with their primary sexual organ. They always imagine the penis as something extraneous, like a faucet, whereas a man thinks of his penis as part of himself, yet self-willed and even disobedient. Similarly, men usually dream of 'pregnancy' as nothing but enormous fatness, with no awareness of a separate life stirring inside them.

Here's the pregnancy-and-birth dream of a 26-year-old car hire receptionist from Denver, Colorado:

I didn't understand that what was happening to me was a dream – not at first anyhow. I was lying down, and I thought I was simply lying in bed waiting to go to sleep. But the lights were very bright, and they were shining in my eyes. I said to my roommate, Terry: 'Switch off the lights, Terry, they're shining in my eyes.' But she didn't answer. Then there was a doctor and a nurse standing next to me. I can't recall the doctor's face, but I can never recall the faces of people I see in my dreams. I can remember his white jacket, and some kind of stethoscope thing that was hanging around his neck. The nurse was wearing a nurse's cap, but she was topless, with small wobbly breasts, and I can remember thinking that they must be so short of hospital staff these days they were roping in topless dancers.

The doctor told me to lift my nightgown. Even though I couldn't see his face, I had the feeling he was rather handsome and attractive. He told me to raise my legs up in the air, and he clamped my ankles to the walls with kind of chrome bracket things that pinched my skin. They started to shine lights between my legs – big, powerful lights that dazzled me. Then they started to discuss my pussy, and the doctor stroked it with his finger while he was talking. They were saying things like 'She has a lot of juice down there,' and 'The skin's very pink,' and 'Do you think she's been fucked a lot?' The doctor started to stroke my pussy with very quick, light strokes, and they started discussing the way my pussy lips were swelling up when I was turned on. I tried to twist around, because I knew I was going to have an orgasm if he went on stroking me like that, and I was embarrassed to have an orgasm with all those doctors and nurses actually staring at my pussy while I did.

But then everything was different. I was sitting on a park bench in Denver, and it was a very windy day. I was wearing a hospital blanket wrapped around my shoulders. I knew that the result of the examination was that I was pregnant, and I was going to have a baby in nine months' time. My stomach was already swelled up, as if I was nearly ready to give birth straightaway, and I could feel the baby kicking and moving inside me. I put my hand on my stomach and felt the way its feet pushed out, and I felt such love for it that I can't even tell you. It was mine. It didn't matter who the father was. Any man could be the father, but this baby was mine, and we were close together like no two people could ever be. I thought to myself that a man can stick his cock inside you, and think that that's the closest that two people can ever be, but your baby is completely inside you — cock, legs, head, body, and arms, and you don't come any closer than that.

I knew I had to hurry to get to the hospital in time. I could feel all these spasms. I tried to run across the road to catch a bus, but the bus didn't wait. It was growing dark, and I was only wearing a hospital blanket. Someone had dropped thousands of glass marbles all over the sidewalk, and I was terrified I was going to slide over and lose the baby. I lay on my side on the sidewalk in case I fell, and a male nurse or a doctor came and lay down beside me. He started to kiss me and nuzzle my neck, and he rubbed his cock up against me and breathed in my ear. I knew that this was the new way of natural childbirth, where the father kind of joins in. He has to make love to his wife while she's giving birth, and that helps her to produce the baby.

I could feel my baby inside me like an orgasm that wouldn't quite come. I held on to my ankles and shut my eyes. I felt as if I was drowning in the sidewalk. I knew there were hundreds of people watching me, but I was too involved in giving birth to my baby to be embarrassed. The baby was kicking and jumping, and it seemed to be growing bigger and bigger the whole time. A priest was kneeling by my head, and he was holding his cock in his hand. I knew that he must be the father, so I kissed the top of his cock, and two drops of holy water came out of the end of it.

Then the baby started to come out of me. It was a sensational feeling. I was worried it was going to get all gritty and dirty on the sidewalk, but someone picked the baby up for me. I was sweating like crazy, and I kept having orgasms. They showed me the baby, and it had bright blue eyes. It smiled at me, and I thought, 'It looks just like my father. I'd better call him up and tell him.'

I know the dream went on after that, but that's all I can remember.

Although this dream seems to be little more than a prenatal examination, followed by an extremely speedy period of gestation and a birth, it is thick with implications and images, and would take many hours of intensive interpretation to unravel. Even then, I suspect that much of it would remain a mystery. Pregnancy is an extremely complicated emotional issue, and many of the major anxieties of motherhood emerge in this one dream. The role of the father, the relationship between mother and child, the ambivalent feelings about giving birth in front of spectators. At the same time, there is no doubt that this is a sexual and sometimes erotic dream, and that she thinks of her childbearing as an integral part of her love making. For a woman who conceives, the act of love is not completed nor whole until the baby is actually born (hence the close comparison between birth and orgasm). The man, on the other hand, has completed his duty the moment he has ejaculated his sperm. This particular dream makes the interesting point that a man could try and think of pregnancy and birth as an ongoing act of love in which he is still involved, and the idea of having sex during parturition – while impossible in practical terms – is a way of expressing that involvement.

While we're on the subject of birth dreams, it's worth mentioning those not uncommon pregnancy dreams in which women are worried that they are going to give birth to a dead or deformed baby or some kind of monster. This is a very familiar fear even in waking life, and there is no need to worry that it's prophetic. The dream might have some relevance as far as your marriage or sexual relationships are concerned. A woman whose marriage is shaky may dream of a dismembered baby, for example – or, as

Dr Faraday pointed out, a racially prejudiced girl may dream of giving birth to animals. One girl even wrote me a letter describing a dream in which she had produced twin bicycles, which the midwife and doctor promptly requisitioned for an acrobatic cycling display. It turned out that the dream was simply an unconscious expression of her dislike for her doctor's psychoanalytical ideas. The phrase 'trick-cyclist' for 'psychiatrist' had filtered into her mind, and gotten tangled up in her dream.

There is so much exhibitionism involved in birth-and-pregnancy dreams that it's natural to look at public nudity dreams next. Many people, both men and women, have sexual dreams of appearing in front of others with no clothes on, and their dreams have several different interpretations. The most common interpretation is that they are anxious about being exposed in public, sexually or emotionally or in any other way. Then there is the possibility that they want to show their real sexual selves, instead of hiding behind their 'persona' – Jung's word for their outward façade. Often, the reaction of the public to the dreamer's nakedness is a vital clue, since the 'public', if they are not identifiable individuals, may represent what the dreamer herself thinks about what she is doing.

Women's nudity dreams tend to differ in several basic ways from men's nudity dreams, however. Women are generally happier with the idea of displaying their naked bodies than men (depending on the circumstances and the audience), and they seem to feel freedom and release more frequently than they feel embarrassment. They will feel embarrassed in dreams when their clothing isn't quite right – their tights have runs in them or their panties won't stay up. But when they're completely nude, or deliberately dressed in a way which shows off their breasts, they appear to feel reasonably at ease – although often excited.

* * *

This is the nudity dream of a 19-year-old trainee teacher from New York:

I dreamed that I was taking a class of adolescent boys and girls, and that I was trying to teach them about rainfall and relative humidity and stuff like that. The only trouble was, I was nude, and the pupils were much more interested in looking at my body than they were in their lessons. I didn't feel embarrassed. I knew that I was older than them, and I was in charge of them, and because of that I could do anything I liked. I could dress any way I liked, and if I wanted to be nude, then I'd be nude. Besides, I didn't know where my clothes were, and I had the feeling I must've left them at home.

Some of the boys in the class were naked, too, and they were masturbating quite openly. I once watched through the crack in the bedroom door while my older brother masturbated, and I guess I was visualizing that all over again. They were dropping their come all over the floor, these kids, and I was trying not to step in it.

Then the girls were naked, too, and they were masturbating. I knew that they were masturbating because of me. I was turning them on. Then they were all laughing because they were coming.

I don't quite know what happened next, but I was running along the school corridor looking for someplace to dress. As I ran along, my boobs bounced up and down, and I could feel them in my dream. In the distance, I could see some of the older teachers coming along, and I knew that if they saw me naked — well, I'd be in a whole mess of trouble.

I hid in an empty room. It wasn't a classroom — in fact, it wasn't even part of the school. It was the sitting room of an apartment I used to share when I first left home. My mother was sitting there doing macrame. I asked her what she was making, and she said 'Tangles.' I had to hide behind the sofa so that she wouldn't see I was nude.

I suddenly realized that one of the boys in my training class was right next to me, hiding under the sofa itself. It was absolutely impossible, because the sofa was only an inch off of the floor, but somehow he had managed to squeeze underneath it. He's a boy called Mark, and he's very good-looking for a fourteen-year-old schoolboy. He came out from under the sofa and lay underneath me and started kissing and fondling my breasts. I tried to tell him to stop it, but then I thought it would be okay. He wouldn't tell anyone, and what was the difference between a lover of twenty and a lover of fourteen? Only six years.

He pushed himself down until his face was right between my legs. I gripped his head in my thighs, and he started to lick my pussy with his tongue. There were blue marks on his tongue, which must've been ink. I held open my pussy for him, and let him push his nose right up inside me. I could see his eyes staring at me through my own pubic hair. It was so real, this dream, I could even feel his teeth nibbling my asshole.

Then we were trying to make love on a long kind of skateboard. I knew I had to reach my climax before we skated around the corner, because then we'd arrive in the playground, and everybody would see us making love. Then everything changed again and I was trying to get into my apartment, but the key wouldn't fit. I was still nude, and I could hear voices of people coming closer. I struck a pose, and I thought to myself, 'Maybe they'll think I'm a pin-up, and go away.'

As in most erotic dreams, there are other sexual themes in this one apart from public nudity. Masturbation, intercourse, and sex with children. But it is the theme of nudity that weaves all these other aspects of the dream together. The girl is trying to give voice in her dream to urges and desires that she has obviously felt several times in waking life, but which she has quickly suppressed.

She is dreaming about her own sexual identity – which at the age of 19 is just beginning to acquire some form and maturity – and she is also dreaming about the sexual interest she feels for her boy pupils. Teachers are not officially supposed to feel that way, but remember that there's only six years between this teacher and her boys, and that she's new to the experience of having twenty or thirty people sitting and watching her so attentively. She feels flattered, she feels proud of herself (hence the admiring masturbation from both boys and girls), and she feels sexy. She is a little worried what officialdom may think (the anxiety about older teachers discovering her nudity), but her dream is surprisingly free of worry and stress and is basically a celebration of her new-found womanly sex. According to several dream dictionaries, dreams of spilled ink are said to foretell the happy conclusion to a long-standing problem.

Erotic dreams about lesbian relationships often worry their dreamers. But remember that the dreaming mind doesn't always share the same inhibitions as the waking mind, and so the idea of kissing or making love to other women may not necessarily offend it. Dreams are far more visual and far less verbal than waking thoughts, and if you feel affection for another woman, it is more likely to appear in your dream as a kiss, rather than the spoken words 'I like you.' Anyway, just because your social conditioning makes you doubtful about sexual love for other women, that doesn't mean for a moment that it's harmful, or that, deep down in your subconscious, you don't sometimes feel such love. We all have both masculine and feminine elements in our makeup, and so there's nothing unusual about feeling a twitch of interest in a pretty or seductive girl.

Remember, too, that the girl you are having sex with in your dream may actually be you yourself. Many so-called lesbian dreams are in fact narcissistic dreams, in which you are showing yourself how much you love your own mind and body. One girl told me that she had a whole series of dreams in which she gave herself cunnilingus (licking her own vulva) and Professor Calvin S. Hall, in his book *The Individual and His Dreams*, mentions two cases of men who dreamed they were sucking their own penises.

Here is a lesbian dream from a 35-year-old divorcee from Richmond, Virginia:

In my dream, I'm a member of a showgirl troupe called The Zizzers, or some crazy name like that. There's probably around a dozen of us, and we're all dressed in silvery-green satin drum majorette's uniforms. Jackets, with epaulets. Tall peaked hats, little pleated skirts, silver satin panties, white boots. We're waiting in a tent someplace, and I look out of the tent-flap across the fields, and I can see dark thundery skies in the distance and trees blowing in the wind, and I know that this is all happening a long time ago, like 1923.

One of the other showgirls comes up to me and asks me how she looks. She's very beautiful. She has big green eyes, and thick curly brown hair, and those real heavy sexy lips. I say she looks fine. But she stays with me, and says, 'How do I *really* look?' I look around and she's holding up her skirt so that I can see her panties. They're shiny and very small — in fact they're so small that I can see her pubic hair, and the sides of her pussy bulging out from the sides of her panties. For some reason, it turns me on, and when she drops her skirt and walks away again, I feel I want to see more.

We all have to climb aboard a strange trailer that's like a kind of spaceship on rails. It's very difficult to climb up the ladder, and the entrance is sealed off with tight rubbery curtains, so you have to force your way through. The curtains are greasy, so you can slip inside the trailer more easily. Inside the trailer is where the girls can undress, and we start chattering and taking off our clothes. Several times naked girls brush their nipples against me, and I feel a surge of real excitement. I try not to look, but I can't help noticing their bare bottoms and their pussies and their breasts. All of the girls are beautiful — blondes, brunettes, and everything, and I know that I'm just as beautiful as they are.

I see the gorgeous girl who came up to me in the tent. She's still wearing her uniform. I walk over and start to unbutton her jacket. Her breasts are bare underneath, and I can almost feel the way they bounce when I undo all the buttons. I take off her skirt, and then I run my hand inside her panties, and start to finger her pussy. It's wet and hot, and she throws back her head and parts her mouth and holds me close. Her bare breasts press against my bare breasts, and I feel so secure and happy. Her hand works its way between my thighs, and starts to touch me up. She seems to have a way of pulling my clitoris that no one else has ever discovered, and I love her so much that I'm almost in tears.

Then we're dressing up again, but this time we're not in the showgirl troupe anymore. We seem to be walking across the plaza outside the John Hancock building in Chicago, which is where my cousin lives. I look up at the John Hancock building, and the beautiful girl whispers something obscene in my ear, and I can't think of anything but how much I want to stay with her. I wonder if it's possible for women to get married. She's wearing a real elegant brown tweed suit, with a 1920s hat, and an alligator pocketbook under one arm. She's so erotic.

Next we're in a corridor someplace. There's the sound of heavy rain outside, but inside it's warm. I'm bending over, touching my toes, and the beautiful girl has got her head under my skirt, and she's pulled down my panties at the back, and she's thrusting her tongue up my anus. She sticks it in right up to her teeth, and she's working one hand into my pussy. The whole hand, diamond rings and all. She's cutting my pussy to shreds with her rings, but I'd do anything for her. She whispers, under my skirt, that her name is Astrid, and she wants me to meet her that night and have sex with her.

I reach around and hold her hand, but when I draw her hand towards me, it's just a living hand that isn't attached to anything. Her tongue is still inside my anus, but the rest of her has disappeared. I look on the wall of the corridor, and I can see her in a photograph of a street in Norfolk, walking across the street in a white hat and a zig-zag black-and-white dress. I push my bottom muscles, and squeeze her tongue out on to the palm of my hand. I stare at it, so sadly, and know that it's all I have left of her. I woke up with my eyes full of tears.

You don't have to look too far to find the principal motivations for this particular dream. The dreamer, a 35-year-old divorcee, had been living on her own since her divorce, and was beginning to feel both frustrated and lonesome. She was dreaming about sex — but she didn't want it from men, in whom she had (temporarily, at least) lost faith. This made her much more receptive to the friendship and sexual attraction of other girls. There is a certain amount of idealistic wish-fulfillment in this dream — the fantasy of a perfect sexual relationship with no complications, no possibility of pregnancy, and no worries about divorce. It is even set in the 1920s, an era that is dim and distant enough to seem romantic and carefree. But in the end, she understands even in her dream that such a relationship cannot exist, and the erotic Astrid vanishes from sight.

Again, there are many erotic images and undertones in this dream which demand closer scrutiny. There are obvious ones – like the vaginal entrance to the showgirls' trailer. There are more subtle ones – like the sound of heavy rain and the photograph of Norfolk. And why Astrid? These are mysteries that only the woman herself can satisfactorily solve.

When we get into erotic dreams of incest, we are heavily into Freudian territory. Oedipus and Electra complexes, ogres and terrible mothers, kings and queens. There is no doubt at all that young girls can get sexually hung up on their daddies, and that brothers and sisters do play doctors and nurses. But the dream and the fact are somewhat different. Although the American Humane Association has recorded 832,000 cases of incest over the past fifteen years – of which nearly three quarters were father-daughter incest – they mostly derived from a specific type of home background. What provoked the incest was not so much the daughter's dream of having sex with her father as the father's dream of having sex with his daughter. In a preponderance of cases, the incestuous father was old-fashioned, domineering, and possessive. He was a reliable provider for his family, and that was usually why his wife managed to be looking the other way when he possessed his daughter. But he was eccentric – one father apparently used to walk about naked with a lighted candle, saying that anyone who looked at him would drop dead. And he was lacking in sexual confidence – he found it easier to get his extramarital oats on the home farm than risk the scorn of strange women.

Unless your own father fits this description, the chances of actual incest occurring are zero. You may be dreaming about your father as a man to whom you are sexually attracted (and it's worth thinking about incest dreams as plainly as this before you start trying to think of dear old Dad as a Freudian symbol). He was, after all, the first man of whom you were ever aware, and it's hardly surprising that his maleness played an important part in the development of your attitude towards men and sex in general. Don't worry about it. Enjoy the dream and just be thankful that the old man doesn't stroll around with lighted candles.

Having said this, it is also possible that your dreams of sexual relations with your father or brother may symbolize some conflict between your family life and your sexual life. What it is will depend on how your lover appears in your dream, and what problems you are personally facing. Your father may be an archetypal dream image for authority and strength, and your brother may represent family affection. It is not unusual for women to have dreams in which their husbands or lovers become confused with their fathers or brothers, and these dreams simply show that the women are transferring their love from within their family to a new family of their own.

Here's an incest dream from a 22-year-old fashion model from New York:

I dreamed my father and I were having lunch at the seafood bar at the Plaza. I knew it was there because there's a black guy with sideburns who serves behind the counter that I recognized. My father was having the fried oysters. I was having a strange kind of a fish that I didn't recognize. It was flat and blue, and I had the feeling that every time I turned my head away, it opened one eye and stared at me. But when I turned back, it closed its eye and pretended to be dead and cooked.

My father was looking very handsome and young. He was wearing a new aftershave. I asked him what it was and he said Ballyhoo, which I guess was a dream thing for Balenciaga. Maybe not, I don't know. My father was speaking very seriously to me, although I couldn't hear what he was saying too well, and I was worried about my fish. But I looked at him every now and then, and I thought he looked very attractive.

In some strange way, I managed to reach down and slide my hand up the leg of his pants. I don't know whether he noticed what was going on or not. I thought that the drapes looked very tatty in the seafood bar, and I wondered what they were made out of. My arm went all the way up my father's pants leg, and I suddenly touched his penis. I had never consciously thought of my father *having* a penis before, and it was quite a shock. Like somehow you never think about your own mother's vagina. His penis was stiff, and seemed to come halfway down his thigh. I gripped it tight in my hand and rubbed it once or twice. I leaned across the table and whispered, 'Father – do you want to fuck me?'

As soon as I said that, the whole scene seemed to change. We were lying on the floor in a different restaurant, halfway under one of the tables. My father was naked. He had gray curly hair on his chest, and gray pubic hair as well. He was trying to get on top of me. I couldn't get my panties down because they were knotted up in a weird kind of way, and so my father had to cut a slit in them with a table-knife. The carpet under the table was very dusty and I started to sneeze.

My father finally managed to wedge his body under the table and bring his penis in line with my vagina. I held his penis in my hand, and guided it towards my vagina. It gave me a strange sensation to think that this same penis had created the vagina it was about to go into, and if I had a baby by my father, I might create another vagina, and so on and so on. It reminded me of those ivory balls within ivory balls within ivory balls.

As soon as I started thinking about ivory balls, we were someplace else, on the deck of the boat my father had rented for fishing when we spent a few months in Florida. I guess the ivory reminded me of shark's teeth and jaws and fishbones. My father was on deck, fishing. He was wearing a life jacket, but that was all. His penis was erect, and the fishing line seemed to be coming out of the hole in the end of his penis, making the same whirring noise as a reel.

Then I was outside my parent's bedroom in Rochester, spying through a crack in the door. I could see into the dressing-table mirror, and I could see my father's bottom and his penis going in and out of a girl's vagina. Pink, hairy vagina. Then I began to understand that it was *my* vagina, and I was watching my father having sex with me. The situation totally confused me, and I had to stop looking. But I stood outside that door, wondering if I ought to go in and watch my father fucking me, or whether something dreadful would happen if I did. I opened the door, and there was a strange girl, not me at all, and she was milking my father's penis into a kind of hospital cup. She looked up and shook her head, and I took that to mean that she thought he was old, and may not live very much longer.

There are plenty of images and symbols in this girl's dream which, when interpreted, will help her to understand her sexual attitude toward her father more exactly. But, even though she was disturbed by the dream, it is obviously nothing to worry about. She was simply dreaming about her father as an attractive man whom she knew rather well, instead of dreaming about him as nothing but a father. Her confusion about her own identity towards the end of the dream indicates that, even in her sleep, she had doubts and anxieties about sleeping with him. And her unconscious – the 'strange girl' – reminded her that her father was a man of an older generation, and not a suitable lover. Fish, which ancient dream books invariably interpreted as a symbol of sex, put in a strong appearance. So do balls and knives and knots – all of which are susceptible of sexual interpretations.

Dreams of sadistic or masochistic sexual behavior are less cozy. By sadism and masochism I don't mean the ordinary day-to-day domination and submission that occur in every sexual relationship. I mean the compulsive erotic pleasure that some people derive from inflicting pain or having it inflicted on them. Although dreams of sado-masochism are not as common as dreams of intercourse or marriage, they certainly rate a position in the top ten erotic dreams. Many women dream of being punished and hurt, and getting a sexual kick out of it. It's easier, of course, than being punished or hurt in real life, because there's no real pain. As Monique von Cleef once told me, lots of people fantasize about being whipped or tortured, and they can turn themselves on by doing it; but when they experience the pain for real, the last thing they're thinking about is sex.

Don't think that women are the only ones who have sexual dreams about being disciplined. Men have them, too. But there are notable differences between the masochism dreams of men and the masochism dreams of women. Men tend to dream of very ritual punishments (just as real, daytime male masochists are aroused by ritual clothing, ritual procedures, ritual pain). Women prefer more spontaneous and vigorous mistreatment. They enjoy the feeling that they can be 'roughly used' by any man who cares to take them. What many women seem to find arousing about *The Story of O* is that O has to be available for anyone at anytime, without any choice in the matter. They are less aroused by the fetishistic trappings, such as the rings piercing O's vaginal lips, the chains, and the whips.

This is a beautiful masochistic dream from a 27-year-old Carolina housewife. When I say 'beautiful', I mean that it has all the richness and color of women's erotic dreams at their most imaginative.

I dreamed that my apartment was full of strange, silent men. There were eight or nine of them, and they were all tall and quiet, and dressed in scaly black leather uniforms. Some of them wore goggles so that you couldn't see their faces. They seemed to spend all their time sitting around my kitchen table, talking softly to themselves so that I couldn't hear what they were saying, and playing a kind of dice game.

At first I tried to ignore them, but then one of them spoke to me, and although I couldn't understand his language, I got the impression that he wanted me to wash the kitchen floor. I filled up a bucket with soapy water, and I tucked my dress up into my panties, and then I got down on my hands and knees and started to scrub. The men looked at me from time to time, but mostly they ignored me. I was wearing stockings and a garter belt for some reason, and they were soaked with foamy water. My hair was hanging loose, and I felt really bedraggled.

Just as I was scrubbing around the legs of the table, one of the men lifted his foot and pointed it towards me. I looked up at him, but he had goggles and leather scales over his face, so I couldn't see who he was. But I knew what he wanted me to do. I had to take the round black toe of his shoe into my mouth and suck it, just to show him that I was his servant. The shoe tasted salty and it felt rubbery in my mouth, and I thought I was going to be sick. I could hear music somewhere. A radio was playing 'Nashville Cats'. Then the man forced his boot right down my throat, and I almost drowned in salty saliva.

Two more men stood up and one of them emptied my bucket right over my head. They pressed me face down against the flooded floor, with their feet on my back. Then another man pushed my legs apart with his foot, pulled open my panties at the back and wedged the big bar of green kitchen soap up my bottom. It gave me an awful pain, as if I wanted to go to the toilet but couldn't.

The kitchen was full of colored smoke, all colors of the rainbow, and I wondered if anyone was smoking grass. There was music playing again, the kind of music that's so lovely that it almost irritates you. I tried to crawl across the floor, but one of the men was sitting on my back. Even though I couldn't actually see what he was doing, I knew that he had taken his prick out of his leather pants and he was rubbing it in my hair. As soon as I realized that, I felt a warm wet feeling on the back of my head, and his come came sliding down the sides of my face and into my nose.

The scene changed, and I was still lying face-down on the floor, but now I was naked, and I was chained to the deck of a rusty ship. We were sailing to Okinawa, I knew that much. I could hear sailors speaking in Japanese, and there was a warm wind blowing across the deck with the scent of spices. Again there was music, very far away, and I couldn't tell where it was coming from.

The rusty deck was very rough against my body, and it was making me bleed. The Japanese sailors were standing around watching me, and sometimes they spat on my bare body. I wanted desperately to masturbate, but I knew that I would have to bend myself double to do it, and I would scrape myself on the deck and get hurt. It was really painful, but in the end I managed to get one chained-up hand between my legs, and I started to masturbate myself in front of all these sailors. They laughed and jeered at me, but I had my eyes closed, and I was dreaming about the ornamental gardens of a strange place somewhere, with soft pink skies and minarets and spires, and there was a dark man, some kind of prince or adventurer, and he was sitting by a reflecting pool and waiting for me. He would know how hurt and abused I'd been. He would know that I'd been spat on and trodden on, and that men had wiped sperm in my hair and pushed things inside my bottom and my vagina, and that would only make him love me all the more.

I seemed to slip from one dream into the other, and then I was lying in the prince's arms like a baby, and he was soothing me and talking to me. He had a sword, a scimitar, and I drew it out from the scabbard around his waist. It was long and curved and very sharp. I held my left hand out and I sliced all my fingers off, one by one, to show him how much I loved him. It was agony, absolute agony, but he laid me down on the cold dewy grass, and he showed me his prick and his balls. They were studded with diamonds and rubies, because he was a prince. I looked up in the sky and it was full of flocks of birds. I wanted him to flock me, but he said he couldn't, and I didn't know what to do next. Then I found I was talking out loud, and I was awake.

It's often difficult to distinguish between dreams of masochism and dreams of rape. The two themes can frequently appear in the same dream, and be inextricably intermingled. But you can usually distinguish between straightforward rape and straightforward masochism by applying this rule-of-thumb. Rape dreams are mainly concerned with forcible intercourse, and dwell less on the pain and the discomfort and more on the pleasure of a man 'having his way' with you against your will. Masochism dreams, on the other hand, depend for their principal thrill on actual pain and humiliation, and quite often have no scenes of intercourse at all. As I've pointed out before, the erotic excitement that rape and masochism dreams stir up has very little to do with how you'd feel if you actually *were* raped or sexually humiliated.

The Carolina housewife who dreamed this masochistic dream appears to be a stable, outgoing woman with no anxieties or fears to cloud her married life. If she persistently has erotic dreams like this, however, she should start to ask herself a few questions about her sexual relationship with her husband. Is he strong enough, physically and emotionally, to give her the security she wants? Or does she crave someone more domineering and decisive?

She should also ask herself if she has enough confidence in her sexual attractiveness and her talents in bed. Masochists invariably underestimate themselves (just as sadists invariably overrate themselves), and it could be that her dreams are pointing out to her just how much of a doormat she's become. Dreams warn, dreams suggest, dreams clarify. If she takes the trouble to interpret the ins and outs of this erotic dream, she will undoubtedly come across some important pointers to her everyday sexual situation.

Some of the events and images in this dream can be quickly traced to actual sexual events. The boot sucking is an obvious vision of fellatio; the bar of green soap forced up her anus may be a reminder of rectal intercourse, or it may go back even earlier to childhood enemas. Goggles or eyeglasses, according to some dream books, signify a relationship that you no longer want, but only the woman herself can be the final judge of that.

Despite the horrifying contents of this dream, it's not as grave or disturbing as it appears at first sight. Slicing fingers off may be a psychotic business in waking life, but in dreams it's only a way of emphasizing a thought or an idea in visual terms. Nonetheless, it's a dream which should be interpreted soberly, and with a careful eye on its relevance to her marriage, because it could be the kind of warning that deserves serious attention.

It's not at all unexpected that erotic dreams of orgasm should also rate high in women's nocturnal thoughts. Orgasm problems have affected almost every woman at one time or another, and they remain the single largest source of female sexual discontent. Orgasms appear in dreams in strange and different ways. If you have a real orgasm while you're dreaming, the orgasm usually figures in the dream itself. But if you only *dream* that you're having an orgasm, you don't necessarily have one for real.

Dream orgasms can closely resemble your waking orgasms, but often they have an extra ingredient that tells you more about your sexual self than a waking orgasm ever can. You'll see what I mean from the sample dream that follows. Occasionally, though, dream orgasms are nothing like waking orgasms at all, and are represented by odd and random events. One girl told me that she stuck her head in a beehive, and she was convinced in the dream that the act of doing that was 'an orgasm'. Another woman had a dream in which she was flung from the top of a fairground Ferris wheel and landed on the back of a carousel horse. When she touched down, she felt as sexually satisfied as if she'd been having strenuous intercourse with her husband. Orgasm is sometimes represented in dreams by death (Freud called the sexual climax 'the little death'), and at other times by running, falling, or swimming.

This is the orgasmic dream of a 25-year-old theater designer from San Francisco. It is actually an amalgam of two dreams which, in isolation, were difficult to understand, but which together form a coherent and interpretable pattern.

I'm sitting by a stone wall under the shadow of Coit Tower with my boyfriend Eddie, and we're trying to decide whether we ought to go and eat, or whether we ought to stay where we are and wait for some friends of ours to show. Everytime I blink, I get the impression that at least an hour or a half-hour has passed, and the sun's moved around. The whole day seems to get shorter everytime I blink. After just a few minutes, it's evening, and we can see the lights of the city twinkling all around us.

We're driving home in Eddie's car, but the roof of the car keeps pressing lower and lower, until our heads are jammed between the front shelf and the roof. Eddie's worried that the police will see his car this way and arrest us, but we manage to find our way home and climb out of the car somehow. Eddie opens the door, and we slide down a sort of chute into the bedroom. We land on the bed, and for some reason we're so heavy that we can't even raise our heads off the sheets.

Eddie crawls over to me, and starts to blow warm air through my cheesecloth blouse on to my nipples. This makes my nipples stick up, and he pops them right through the fabric. He's beginning to turn me on. I kiss him and ruffle his hair. Then I open his pants, and take out his cock, and I show him this new trick I've taught myself. I can hold his cock between my thighs, and actually make my thighs vibrate. I tell him I can make him come in ten seconds. He laughs and says he doesn't believe me.

I go down on my hands and knees on the bed, and Eddie puts his cock in from behind, and we start to make love like that. The door opens a crack. My mother is standing outside, and she's holding a currant cake in a warm tea towel. She keeps calling my name, and I put my head around the door and talk to her, even though Eddie's still fucking me. I reach behind me, and I open myself as wide as possible, so that Eddie can go deep. My mother says, 'I always had trouble with your father,' and I ask her, 'What kind of trouble?' She's still holding the cake, and she says, 'Cake trouble – I always had cake trouble.'

I ask her what she means, and she says I mustn't worry about it. But she passes the cake around the door. She can't resist peeking around, too, and she sees Eddie fucking me, although I don't want her to.

Eddie's plunging in and out of me real fast. I hold the warm cake against my clitoris, and I start to have an orgasm. I feel as if my forehead has turned into a TV screen, and there are white flashes and blips going through the blackness. Eddie pours his sperm into me 'like Irish coffee,' I think. I feel pleasure all over me, and it's all rising up from the warm cake. I know now that if

I want to have an orgasm every time, I'll have to ask my mother to bring one.

We're in my mother's house, in the kitchen, and I can smell food baking. Eddie is sitting on a three-legged stool at the end of the room. He has a furry jacket on, but otherwise he's naked. His toes are curled up. He's masturbating, with a very serious look on his face. My mother comes in with her hair in curling papers. She doesn't look at Eddie, although I know she disapproves. She starts to cut a large piece of meat on a wooden board, and she asks me to lean forward and watch. It's not a piece of meat at all, but a vagina, and she quietly tells me all about it so that Eddie won't hear. She points out the clitoris, and says I have to put plenty of pepper on it, otherwise I'm always going to be disappointed. It all seems very clear, all this talk about pepper. Eddie comes up to me and slides his cock into me without my mother noticing at first. But when she does, she comes around the table with a handful of red-hot pepper, and she rubs it furiously into my clitoris. It's just like having a mouthful of chilis, only right on my clitoris instead. It's hot and itchy and it turns me on. I start to twitch and shake and shudder, and Eddie grabs my shoulders from behind and he's really ramming it up me, so hard that it's making a sucking noise. I'm all tensed up like a bowstring. I lift my legs in the air until they're braced against the kitchen table, and I'm clenching my fists and screwing my eyes tight shut. I think I'm going to die, or burst, or something. Then the orgasm hits me like a crack in a log of wood. I scream out loud because I don't know whether it's beautiful or horrible.

Although the girl did not actually experience orgasm for real during either of the two dream orgasms, they were very realistic climaxes. Often, dream orgasms are accompanied by smiles of happiness and pleasure, but as Kinsey once remarked: 'Unresponsive wives who attempt to make their husbands believe that they are enjoying coitus fall into an error because they assume that an erotically aroused person should look happy and pleased and should smile and become increasingly alert as he or she approaches the culmination of the act. On the contrary, an individual who is really responding is as incapable of looking happy as the individual who is being tortured.'

I should explain that this particular girl had been having severe psychological difficulties in achieving orgasm, and although her problem had been partially eased by therapy, she still wasn't achieving the kind of orgasm rate that Masters and Johnson consider to be minimally satisfying – fifty percent. She wasn't married, although she had lived with her boyfriend for two years as man and wife.

The orgasm problem may have been caused by her unconscious inhibitions about 'living in sin' – inhibitions which the permissive attitudes of her friends didn't allow her to voice or admit. But she did not want to get married simply to overcome orgasmic dysfunction. She wanted to marry when her career had developed further, and she had had the opportunity to travel more and meet more people. If she married at all.

Her erotic dreams indicate that she would be wise not to marry in the specific hope of scoring better orgasms. Any girl who dreams that she needs to press warm cakes or red-hot peppers to her clitoris is obviously lacking one important thing – adequate external stimulation from her lover. Whether it's physical or emotional arousal that Eddie isn't giving her, he's not doing what he ought to be doing to get his lady going. Other problems in their relationship are highlighted by these dreams, too. The slowly-sinking car roof may indicate a feeling of being trapped and oppressed. The disapproval that her mother shows for Eddie may really indicate that the more conformist and traditional part of the girl's own personality doesn't think very much of him.

In sum, this is the kind of orgasm dream that can give you sound warnings about your sexual relationships and attitude.

Last of all, I want to look at erotic dreams of feminine

liberation. These are mainly visited upon women whose consciousness of their own sexual identity is in the process of being raised. But they are interesting as a topical sexual phenomenon, and they clearly illustrate the principal theme of this book: that women's dreams are different and separate from men's dreams, and that through their dreams they can help themselves to solve some of their sexual problems and discover their own sexual identity.

Dreams of sexual freedom are very varied and erratic, and it is hard to pick out a 'typical' liberationist dream. I have chosen the sample dream that follows not because it typifies all liberationist dreams that I have come across, but because it is idiosyncratic and colorful, and shows just how powerful a woman's sense of her sexual individuality can be. It comes from a 23-year-old advertising assistant from New York:

I was walking across a wide beach on a windy day. The sand was white, the sea was shining. I felt alone, and a little lonesome, but mostly happy. I could hear birds crying, and I stood for a long time looking out to sea and wondering about myself and about my life.

Then I saw a man coming towards me across the sea. I could hardly look at him, because the reflection on the water was so bright. He seemed to be traveling in a kind of surf-shell, like a large scallop shell. I was on top of the cliffs now, and I looked down and saw him trudging up the beach, with his head bowed, very slowly. He wended his way up the cliff path. He was wearing gold armor, very highly polished. It took him hours to reach the top of the cliff, and I can remember being worried in case I woke up before he got there.

I was still sitting there when he finally reached the top. He didn't seem to be tired or out of breath. He was tanned, with a curly blond beard. He was good-looking. Just the kind of man I like. He squatted down on his haunches and grinned at me. His armor was just a breastplate. He was wearing sandals, laced up to his knees. But he was naked apart from that, and his long penis was hanging between his legs, next to his dagger and his sword. He had long blond pubic hair that curled around his penis, and he was obviously *goyish*.

He started talking and bargaining the way you see Arabs doing it in bazaars. He said he was going to have sex with me. It was necessary, he kept saying. Once he had done it, he would be able to continue with his work. I said that he looked attractive, and that I agreed to have sex with him. But I wanted him to lie on his back, and I would mount him. He said that was very difficult, and he didn't want it that way. He was a warrior, and warriors never lay on their backs. I explained to him that I never lay on my back either, and I wasn't about to start now.

It was one of those dreams where the scenery seems to change around you without you being aware of it. It reminded me of those old Krazy Kat cartoons, where they're standing in a desert when they're talking about deserts, and standing next to the ocean when they're talking about oceans. And the language we spoke was like that, too. I remember Kat saying: 'Dollin, shooly you ixejjirate.' Everything I said in this dream was in this weird language.

We weren't on top of the cliff anymore. We were sitting in a forest clearing, and we were surrounded by men and women in very elegant suits, sipping highballs, and smoking from long holders. The women were all dressed in feathers and silks and impossible shoes, and they clung around the men like moths.

I shifted myself up towards the warrior, and I gripped his hand. I don't know whether I was really holding my own hand or something, but I could feel his hand as if it was solid flesh. I tried to Indian wrestle him. He was very strong, and he almost pushed my arm flat to the ground, but I spoke to him in our peculiar language, and after a while his arm sank, and I clambered on top of him, pushing him flat on his back on the damp leaves.

His penis was very big, and it was standing up now. I was sitting astride him, and I lifted up my dress, so that my cunt was bare, and I took his penis in both hands and positioned it up against my cunt. Then I lifted both feet off the ground, so that my own weight made me sink right down on to his penis.

I made him make love to me the way I wanted. I had never made love like this before. I set the pace and the rhythm, I decided when we should change position and when we should start working ourselves up towards a climax. I started doing fantastic virtuoso things, like spinning round on his penis like a propeller on an airplane.

I woke up then. I was bitterly disappointed that the dream hadn't continued, but I felt as if an enormous weight had been lifted from off my shoulders. I thought – here's this dream, and it's telling me something. It's telling me that I'm a free person, and what's more than that, I'm a free woman. I'll never forget that dream. It's not often a dream tells you something as important as that.

This wasn't a particularly violent or militant dream. The moment of liberation came from a comparatively cordial hand-wrestle, and a calm argument about who's supposed to sit on top of whom. But some liberation dreams are extremely violent – so violent that they can almost be called sadistic dreams. One girl from Los Altos, California, told me that she dreamed she machine-gunned her father, her brothers, her husband, her lovers, and any male who was unfortunate enough to make an appearance in her dream. She interpreted the machine gun as a phallic symbol, and the meaning of the dream as revenge against men by turning their own deadly weapon on to them, and mowing them down – 'just as the cock mows women down.'

Then there was the liberation dream of a housewife from Ann Arbor, Michigan, who fantasized that she was hunting her husband through the house with a carving knife, threatening to cut his sexual organs off. Or the wife from Wichita, Kansas, who dreamed that she knocked her husband down with his own LTD. Or the girl from New Orleans, who beat her boyfriend insensible with spiked gloves that she'd seen in *Rollerball*.

It's interesting to me that so many women, as part of their liberation, feel it necessary to seek *revenge* on men – quite often with men's own symbols of masculine status and power. I guess there are many women who have something to be vengeful about, but it's a classic lesson of history that no revolution ever achieves genuine liberation for its followers unless they eschew the oppressive methods of the regime they are trying to overthrow. If we have women emasculating men instead of men dominating women, we're sexually no better off.

That's why I like the erotic dream of the advertising assistant from New York, with her Indian wrestling and her warrior in golden armor. Her liberation came when she showed him that she had her own ideas about sex and sexual pleasure, that she was as powerful a character as he was, and that she sought respect *from* him rather than revenge *on* him. I share her regret that the dream didn't carry on longer. I would like to have known what happened after they made love, and how she felt.

The ten dreams you have read in this chapter are all long and detailed dreams, recalled by women who have tried to train themselves to remember as much of their nighttime adventures as possible. When you start recording your own dreams, you'll probably find that you can't remember quite as much as these women have been able to. But as time goes by, and you become more proficient, you'll be amazed at the quality and quantity of dream material that you can bring to mind when you wake up.

In the following chapter, you'll discover how to keep a dream diary, and how to assemble your erotic dreams into meaningful series, all ready for interpretation.

Meanwhile, you have a general idea of how to classify your dreams according to their main themes. This will help to give you some indication of what basic problems or situations are being 'discussed' by your dreams, and where you should begin to look for answers to the mysteries they present you with.

If your sexual dreams do not seem to fit any of the top ten categories we've talked about, try to identify the main theme, and use your own judgement to interpret what relevance it has to your present sexual situation. The connection is usually pretty clear. If it isn't, don't try to force an interpretation on it that you're not really sure about. Put the dream to one side. You'll probably find that, several weeks later, you have another dream that throws some more light on it.

Never be dogmatic about classifying your erotic dreams. The classifications I've given here – rape, orgasm, birth-and-pregnancy, liberation, and all the rest – are simply general guides to help you analyze the detail of the dream, when you are ready to do so, more effectively. If the details are consistently awkward and don't seem to fit the main theme, then you must be prepared to reconsider your original classification. As we've seen, the differences between rape and masochism dreams in terms of images and events are not great, but the implications they hold are poles apart.

Remember always that your erotic dreams are created by you, and that they're not disconnected visitations from goblins and genies. *You* made them, *you* put them together, and so *you* are the best person in the world to understand what they mean. They're relevant to your life and your problems, and as Jung said: 'When we lose our way among the endless details and detached events of the superficial world, what would be more natural than to expect to knock on the door of our dreams and ask for views on those problems which could reorient us toward fundamental human facts. Even if the whole world seems out of joint, that all-pervading quality of the mysterious soul cannot break into pieces.'

Okay, then. It's time for you to gird your mysterious soul, take out your erotic dream diary, and see what strange fish you can catch from the seas of the night.

3

Keeping a Sex Dream Diary

By itself, one erotic dream isn't worth very much – not unless it's one of those rare flashes of dreaming insight that happen about once in a lifetime. You probably haven't managed to remember all of your dream, and what you can remember is probably distorted. Try and describe everything you did yesterday when you were awake, and you'll begin to see just how unreliable your memory can be. Don't get upset, though; mine's just as bad as yours.

Most psychologists and dream researchers agree on the usefulness of recording a series of dreams. As Professor Calvin S. Hall explains: 'When a person begins to keep a record of his dreams, he will not at first recognize any connection of subject matter from one night to the next. The dreams will appear completely dissociated from each other, occurring in a random fashion. As the number of dreams in the record increases, then the dreamer will begin to recognize repetitions, regularities, and consistencies. The same characters, situations, activities and objects, and the same themes repeat themselves.'

There are three main threads of consistency running through your dreams. There is the thread of *absolute constancy* – those images that appear with unfailing regularity even if you keep a dream diary for thirty years. There is the thread of *relative consistency* – the unvarying frequency with which one type of dream image appears in relation to another type of dream image. In other words, you might always dream more about meringues than you dream about settees. Then there is the thread of *developmental regularity* – consistent changes in your dreams which relate to gradual developments and changes in your waking life.

You'd be amazed (and you will be amazed, when you start your sex dream diary) at just how unvarying your dreams really are. When you have a new boyfriend or get married or start a new job or move to a new city, the new people and events that you have come to know will begin to appear in your dreams. But the frequency with which you dream about particular types of people never alters. You will dream about your new boss just as often as your old boss. You will dream about the new men and women you know in *just the same proportion of males to females* as the old men and women you used to know. You will dream about your new apartment no more frequently than you dreamed about your old apartment. The characters and the environment may change, but your dreams remain constant.

Why? And why is this so important?

Well, your dreams remain constant because your personality remains constant. Yours are what Professor Hall calls 'a fairly stabilized organization of personality traits, attitudes, and behavioral patterns.' The desires and anxieties you felt at the age of five will still be with you when you're fifty. There are unalterable factors in your personality that make you the person and the woman you are.

If your dreams remain consistent, that means that they are accurately reflecting the basic you. Although the contents of your dreams may vary superficially, the fundamental themes that run through them will give you vital clues about your sexuality and your character. No other method of self-analysis can tell you so much about yourself so truthfully, because recording your erotic dreams is the only way of coaxing sexual opinions out of yourself when your conscious mind is completely off guard. As any sex researcher will tell you, it is almost impossible to get people to give an honest answer to a sexual question. They are too worried about what the researcher will think of them if they answer too frankly, or just what he'll think of them if they don't answer frankly enough. The bane of most researchers' lives is the people who invent answers because they're trying to be helpful.

But your erotic dreams don't invent answers. They create, but they don't fabricate. They joke, but they don't lie. And if you're honest enough to face what they're telling you, you'll get the truth, and nothing but the truth.

It goes without saying that the more dreams you record in your erotic dream diary, the more accurate your personality readings will eventually be. A girl I talked to when I was preparing *1,001 Erotic Dreams Interpreted*,[1] reported a series of sadomasochistic dreams in which she had imagined her boyfriend burning her with cigarette ends and other Nazi-type tortures. She thought that her unconscious mind was warning her about the possible consequences of her boyfriend's rather chauvinistic attitudes. But, a year later, when she was dating a mild and liberal young man instead, she still had the same kind of dreams. The masochism was within her own personality, and it would have manifested itself in her sexual dreams no matter who she was going out with. But it took two quite lengthy dream records before she was willing to see that fact in perspective.

Don't think that you'll find it any easier to admit the sexual truth that your dreams tell you. In my experience, it takes a whole weight of overwhelming evidence to convince most people that they really do have a sexual personality full of quirks and kinks and moments of failure. It's nice to interpret your sexual dreams if they

[1] Henry Regnery Company, 1976.

keep telling you that you're beautiful and well-adjusted and you have enormous sexual potential — but supposing they tell you that you're something of a sadist when it comes to men, and that you have trouble reaching a climax unless you've got your teeth sunk deep in his shoulder and your nails ripping his back up?

The main thing is not to fret. The whole reason you're analyzing your erotic dreams is to find out the truth about your sex life, and if you know the truth, no matter how hair raising it is, then you're halfway to solving your sexual problems, and more than halfway to discovering the full strength and character of your sexual self.

I had five or six dreams over a period of just over four months, and they all worried the hell out of me. The dream was weird enough the first time I had it, but when I had it again and again I began to think there was something really wrong with me. It was only when I pieced the dreams all together that I realized what they revealed.

It always started the same way. I was lying on some hot dry rocks in the desert in Mexico. I was wearing nothing at all but a black tanga — you know, those little tie-up bikini bottoms. My hair was all spread out over the ground, and I was roasting myself browner and browner.

Then, in the distance, I heard bells, and I could smell incense. A line of six or seven monks were coming down the rocks towards me, ringing a bell and shaking incense from a censer. They were singing Latin chants. They wore dark brown habits, and their faces were covered with cowls. When they saw me, they all stood around, singing and swinging their incense. Their faces were hidden in shadow, and at first I was frightened. Gradually, though, when they didn't make any move towards me, I grew a little bit bolder. I stood up and pranced around them, bouncing my breasts and wiggling my butt.

Then I went right up to one of them, and put my arms around him, and I rubbed my leg up against him. I slipped my hand inside his habit, and I could touch his erect prick. I knelt down on the rocks in front of him, and started sucking and licking his prick — really obscenely, pushing it into my cheeks to make them bulge out, and making all these moaning and drooling noises. When he came, I swallowed some of his sperm, but the rest I held in my mouth, and smeared over my lips. Then I went from one monk to the other, kissing them, and spitting a little sperm into each of their mouths, so they all tasted the sperm of the monk I'd been sucking.

The monks went on singing, and the censer went on smoking, and this made me furious. I remember cursing and swearing and calling them every foul name you can think of. I dashed across like a crazy animal, and tore open one monk's habit, and sank my teeth into his stiff prick like sinking your teeth into a sausage. It tasted delicious – sweet and meaty, like pork. I had to have more, and he stood there, not saying a word, while I knelt between his legs and devoured his whole penis and his balls. I knew that I was addicted now, and that I was going to have to eat more and more pricks, or I'd go mad.

This is an extremely savage and disturbing sadistic dream from a 24-year-old telephone operator from Houston, Texas. What made it even more offensive to her was the mockery it made of religion. She was not what anyone could call devout, but she did attend church regularly, and in waking life the idea of humiliating a member of holy orders was anathema to her. But she needn't have worried. Although the dream does seem on the surface to be sadistic and blasphemous, later variations of it showed that it was not all that it seemed to be.

I dreamed that I'd been attacking the monks, and I had to go and explain what I'd been doing to the Mother Superior of a convent nearby. It was so hot, and the sun was shining so brightly that I could hardly see. There were grapevines growing in the courtyard of the convent, and I could hear cicadas chirping. The Mother Superior was an old woman in a white starched robe. She sat on a plain wooden chair in the middle of the courtyard, and she was sewing a sampler with flowers on it. I still had my mouth full of monks' pricks, and I was trying to chew and swallow it all before she noticed.

She started to ask me questions, very quickly, at the top of her voice, and she hardly seemed to wait for the answers. But as she talked, I began to understand what she was going on about. She was trying to explain that it was no good trying to shock myself or the angel within me, and that it was possible to have sex without any of the problems that I'd been having. She raised her hand, and when I looked around the courtyard I saw that, in every alcove, a young man was standing. Really handsome, and naked, and they all had long heavy pricks, with veins in like twisted trees.

From this additional information, it was possible for this girl to interpret her dreams as an allegory of her own sexual conflicts. She had had an affair with a married man, and although she had basically been happy, she had always had underlying anxieties about the morality of what she was doing. She had spoken to her father about it, and he had sternly suggested that she give up the affair and 'find a respectable young man instead.' Her lover, too, began to express doubts about their relationship.

The appearance of the monks represents her spiritual conscience. As Tom Chetwynd says in his *Dictionary for Dreamers*: 'True to their usual function, dreams try to keep a balance between inner spiritual values and sexuality. Those who make an enemy of the spirit, either by neglecting it or by only accepting its outward form, will have this brought to their attention.'

But, in her dream, this girl realizes that she is not afraid of her conscience. She provokes the monks, and in the end she challenges them to the utmost, by turning them on sexually and by flaunting her sexual freedom in front of them. It is hard to give a definitive interpretation of the prick-devouring scene, but the girl herself thinks that it is not an act of sadistic aggression against the monks. She thinks instead that it's a visual scenario to represent her devouring passion for the married man she loves. She was conscious in the dream that it was *his* sexual organs she was eating, not the sexual organs of strange monks. Some ancient interpretations of cannibalistic dreams suggest that the dreamer is trying to draw sexual power from others by eating their private parts, but this analysis, which is based on the ideas of primitive religions, seems to be inappropriate in this case.

The white-robed Mother Superior appears to be an archetypal dream figure – a matron, a grandmother, a sympathetic adviser. She appears in all kinds of traditional dramas and stories – for instance, as the nurse in *Romeo and Juliet*. She explains to the girl that it might be worth considering leaving her married lover, because she is carrying on the affair partly for the sensational effect she is creating. She points out all the other young men that she could have in her life, without any of the same problems. She is continuing the affair because she loves the man, but also because she is being defiant and slightly scandalous. I was interested in her phrase about 'trying to shock myself or the angel within me,' because it recalled a line in a poem by Lawrence Ferlinghetti: ' "I feel there is an angel in me," she'd say, "whom I am constantly shocking." ' It was a quote from Jean Cocteau originally, but the girl had never in her life read either Cocteau or Ferlinghetti.

There is plenty more meaning stashed away in this dream series, but the point I am making by quoting it at such length is that, by itself, the first dream was confusing and frightening and could easily have been misinterpreted. It needed more information, more images, more dreams about the same subject before the core of its implications became clear. The more dreams you can remember the less likely you are to make a substantial error of interpretation. That is where the erotic dream diary comes into its own.

The greatest single difficulty in interpreting your erotic dreams is catching hold of them in the first place. Although we all have at least half-a-dozen dreams every night – usually more – the percentage of dreams we actually remember is minuscule. Some women don't remember any dreams at all.

Why do we forget our dreams? There are several explanations, and some interesting new theories, but no one has yet come up with the definitive answer. So the best thing you can do is take note of all the ways in which you can improve your erotic dream recall and see if your memory perks up.

There is no question that, if you wake up quickly, you will remember your dreams better than you will if you wake up slowly. Countless laboratory dream tests have shown that volunteers who are jolted from their sleep by a loud noise are more likely to remember their dreams more vividly than those volunteers who were allowed to wake up naturally. So if you have an alarm clock, you can probably recall your erotic dreams quite well — better than if you didn't have one.

Women who find it difficult to remember their erotic dreams usually seem to need more stimulus to wake up (alarm bells, shaking, lights) than women who find it easy to remember their erotic dreams. In other words, it seems less likely that you'll remember your dreams vividly if you're a deep sleeper. You could try going to bed earlier if you're really interested in catching your dreams: by morning, when you often have an hour-long period of dream-filled REM sleep, you may be sleeping less heavily than you would be normally. Therefore, your chances of remembering what goes on may be enhanced.

Your personality may also affect your ability to recall dreams. Psychological tests have indicated that people who can't recall their dreams are often inhibited, conformist, and very self-controlled. It's possible that they are deliberately looking away from their dreams when they're asleep, particularly when their dreams contain unpleasant or frightening events. People who are good at recalling their dreams are usually extroverted, easygoing, and willing to admit their fears and their anxieties.

Freudian analysts believe that if we can't recall a dream, then our mind has deliberately 'repressed' it. We don't want to face up to what the dream has told us, and so it slips away into forgetfulness. As Freud himself said: 'The forgotten part provides the best and readiest approach to the understanding of the dream. Probably that is why it sinks into oblivion.' He found that his own dreams often vanished from his memory, even though he'd taken the trouble to interpret them when he woke up during the night. 'It happens far more often that the dream draws the findings of my interpretive activity back with it into oblivion than that my intellectual activity succeeds in preserving the dream in my memory.'

Experiments by Professor R. Whitman at the University of Cincinnati College of Medicine in Ohio have shown that Freud's notion of dream repression had a lot of truth in it. Several subjects 'failed' to recall sexual or aggressive events in their dreams – particularly to people they thought might understand or see through them. So there is certainly a conscious or unconscious censoring going on in your mind, and if you want to recall the most significant parts of your erotic dreams, you will have to be on your guard against it.

Another reason why we forget our dreams is because our mind is not functioning in the same logical progression when we are asleep as it is when we're awake. That is why it's essential to wake up quickly and promptly and to write down or tape-record your dreams at once.

Before you go to sleep, think to yourself that you are going to try and remember a dream tonight. This doesn't always work, but it helps. Keep your erotic dream diary beside your bed, and make sure you know where to find the lightswitch. Thousands of dreams have drained away down the plughole of forgetfulness while the dreamer struggled to locate the lightswitch. Have a pen handy, too, so that you can write down your dream without delay.

You will find your own best method for writing down your dreams, but I prefer to jot down a quick series of key words that sum up the whole framework of the dream in a matter of seconds. Often, if you try to get into flowery description straightaway, you will find that the latter part of the dream escapes you – and it may well be the most significant part. You're not trying to create a literary masterpiece, all you're trying to do is nail down a very elusive and slippery thought before it wriggles away from you into the night.

Having jotted down your series of key words: 'Plane – thunderstorm – stewardess strips – chimpanzees – bells – Viking – rape,' you can begin to flesh out the dream with details of clothing, conversations, characters, odd events, and images. You won't be able to remember everything, especially at first, but do try and recall any particularly evocative images, any strange or frightening or arousing sights, and any 'nonsense' words or conversations. Often the key to the whole dream rests on one peculiar statement from one of the people in it. A New York secretary had a totally confusing dream about some moving men trying to force a vast settee through her front door. It was only when she had the dream for a third time that she recalled one of the men saying 'Crow pie.' She puzzled over this for days before she suddenly realized that the man had been saying *croupier*. Her boyfriend was a croupier, and she had been worried about having intercourse with him because he was very much bigger than her, physically, and she was afraid of being hurt. The 'vast settee' was a symbolic phallus forcing its way into her 'front door'. Once she knew what the dream was *about*, she knew what it *meant*, but if she had never recalled the words 'crow pie', she would never have discovered what her dream signified. So do try and think of every little quirky phrase, saying, and sign.

Do write down what you think the dream means when you first wake up, and if you have any ideas about which daytime events it might be connected with, then do make a note of those, too. Don't assume that you'll remember anything in the morning, because you won't. Be careful to write down exactly what you dreamed, and don't try to alter it while you write to fit into the kind of shape you think it ought to have had. Don't include anything you can't quite recall, and don't try to make the dream into a 'story' with a beginning, a middle, and an end. No matter how illogical or silly or outrageous the dream may seem, its meaning will stay intact only if you resist the temptation to rationalize it into a movie scenario.

It's possible to provoke yourself into having erotic dreams. This can be useful if you're trying to compile a dream series about your current sexual situation, and you're rather short of vivid material. I can't guarantee that the dreams will all be relevant to the situation you want to know more about since some of them will obviously reflect the stimulation you have used to evoke them. But you will probably find a few appropriate images and scenes floating out of your erotic unconscious, and any erotic dream is better than no erotic dream.

Some ways to put your mind into the right kind of mood for erotic dreaming are as follows: read a very sexy book before you go to sleep, preferably a porno magazine with bright, memorable and very erotic pictures; masturbate to the brink of orgasm but then stop; make love to the brink of orgasm but then stop; think about an erotic situation you would like to be in, and draw it; think about a very sexy costume you would like to wear, and draw yourself wearing it; draw an enormous male organ.

Drawing is an important aid to provoking erotic dreams. It firmly imprints visual images on your mind — images which may surface a few hours later in your dreams. As far as anyone can tell, this system may not always work, but enough women have recalled enough of the images they thought about before they went to sleep to make it worth a try.

Here is an excerpt from the six-month erotic dream diary of a New York publishing assistant who tried various ways of stimulating herself sexually before she went to sleep. In each case, she states what she did to provoke erotic dreams, and whether she thinks it worked or not. Certain identifying names have been excised from the diary to protect the girl's identity, but otherwise you're reading it here just as it was written by her:

April 8: Before I went to sleep, lay in the dark for ten or fifteen minutes, gently pressing thighs together and thinking about sexual things, like being in a harem — always a favorite fantasy of mine. Had a long dream that didn't start off sexy, but seemed to get sexier as it went along.

I was sitting in a railroad car, and the train was sliding quite fast through the night. I tried to peer out of the window, but all I could see was lights. A conductor went past, and I asked him where we were. He said, 'Saucepan lids,' and moved on down the corridor.

The seats of the train were hairy and rough, like sitting on dark brown sacks. They were quite comfortable, but they were itchy. I was only wearing a thin dress and white stockings, and the hairs prickled through the material. I knew I wasn't wearing panties. I had an idea that I might have left them in the dining car. I seemed to recall an earlier dream in which I didn't have a napkin in the railroad dining car, and I'd had to wipe my mouth with my panties instead.

I was sitting in the compartment when the door slid back and a tall man in a very expensive gray suit came in. He lifted his hat to me, and sat down opposite. He opened a newspaper and began to read, and he also started smoking a big cigar. I sat there trying to read his newspaper for a while, but somehow the words didn't seem to make any sense. I can't recall any particular words now, but I know there were some real strange ones.

I wanted to attract the man's attention, so I opened my thighs and lifted my skirt, so that my pussy was exposed. Then I gave a polite cough. I thought perhaps he would look up and see me. But he just went on smoking and reading his newspaper.

I coughed some more, and he still didn't look up, so I got off my seat, lifted my skirt right up around my waist, and climbed on to his lap. I undid his fly, reached my hand inside, and started to masturbate his cock. He still kept his hat on. There was a ticket of some kind stuck in the hatband, and I made a mental note to myself to steal it when we were through.

To my surprise, the man looked up and whistled. There were more men out in the corridor. They came inside. There were three of them. One was tall and looked Swedish. The other two were quite dark and could have been Italians. They were all smart like the first man, and they smelled of flowery perfumes. One of them was carrying a green tissue parcel, and I knew intuitively that it was 'a gift for the Wobblies'.

The men opened their pants, and their cocks stuck out like pink sticks of rock candy. I was kneeling on the legs of the first man, and the other men clustered around me and started rolling their cocks all round my thighs and pussy and stomach. I took as many cocks in my hands as I could, and I masturbated them all, until the come started flying through the compartment like snow.

I heard a train door bang somewhere outside, and I knew that someone important had escaped into the night. I tried to go after them, but the men pressed me face down on the seat and raped me, one after the other. I was worried that the pattern of the seat would mark my face, and everybody would know what had happened to me. Someone was out there in the cold night. But I began to have a whole series of orgasms. I was rolling about on the seats and the floor, sobbing. People came around to stare at me, and I clung on to their legs and shoes, still sobbing, and still having these huge orgasms. I woke up then. There were tears in my eyes, and my bed was all twisted up.

April 23: I tried to give myself sex dreams for several nights, without being able to. At least, I couldn't remember any of them. But tonight I did manage to remember something. I took a copy of *Playboy* to bed with me. I borrowed it from my boyfriend. There were some scenes from sexy movies in there, and I gently masturbated while I looked at them. I started off by having dreams about the movies, but gradually they changed into my own dreams.

In the main dream, I was walking through the snow in the fields near my mother's house in New Hampshire. I was wearing a huge white fur coat, and long knee-length leather boots. The sun was very low in the sky, and it was bright orange. It seemed like February.

In the distance, I could see someone waving to me. I tried to run over to see who it was, but the snow was too deep, and I couldn't run properly. My legs seemed to be stuck together. But then I was trudging through a small pine wood. I know it was a pine wood because there was a strong scent of pine. Someone else was walking in the wood, and I could hear branches cracking. They were chasing me, whoever they were. I started to walk faster, but if I walked faster, I began to excite myself – sexually, I mean. I was nude beneath my fur coat, and the coat was buckled together with a very complicated clasp. The faster I ran, the more this clasp seemed to slip open, and it was too compli-cated for me to stop and do it up.

After awhile, I slowed down and let my pursuers catch up with me. I thought I might as well get it over with. Whatever they were going to do, it couldn't be anything like as bad as running through this wood. I turned around to face them. It was my brother Mark and one of the men who work at my office, Dennis. He's nothing special, and I've never even noticed him before. He helps pack up books and send out orders and menial stuff like that.

They each caught hold of an arm. Mark said to Dennis that he knew how to tie me up, because I was his sister. They found a tree that leaned over at an angle of around forty-five degrees. They pushed me back so that I was leaning backwards over it, and then they buckled my arms and legs around it with leather belts. So I was strapped to this tree, with my fur coat wide open, and my brother and this Dennis stood either side of me. They had rough leather britches on, which they opened up and took their cocks out of. Their cocks were strange – all covered in dark fur, like sealskin. They brushed my breasts with their furry cocks, and when they began to let them run down my body, I realized their cocks weren't real cocks at all, but live creatures like rats. I was terrified they were going to let one of them run up inside my pussy.

I felt a wriggling feeling down between my legs, and I looked down just in time to see one of the rats slithering up inside me. It felt very sexy, but at the same time I was terrified. I took hold of its tail — I can't remember how I got my arms free — and I tried to tug it out of me. It didn't want to come, so I tugged harder and harder. Then I realized the only way to get it out would be to masturbate very hard, until I had a climax, and when I had a climax, it would pop out. I sat astride the tree with my legs apart, rubbing my pussy like mad, and at last the rat disappeared.

My brother spoke very loud in my ear. He called my name. He said: 'Now you're in for it.' He pushed me face down in the snow. It was intensely cold but it wasn't wet. My brother fell on top of me. I could feel his warmth and his weight. Then I felt his cock against my pussy, and the beautiful feeling as it pushed its way in. Then he spoke my name again — so loud that I woke up. I looked around, but no one had spoken to me. It had seemed so loud, I couldn't believe that no one had actually said it.

May 6: This time, I tried more obvious stimulation. I bought a vibrator from a store not far away from my office. I was kind of embarrassed about buying it, but the woman behind the counter didn't turn a hair. I took it home and tried it out before I went to sleep. I'm not sure whether I liked the vibrator or not, but it certainly aroused me sexually. The dreams I had were not at all clear. There were several vivid images, but they were extremely disjointed. I had to resist the temptation to join them all together into a story that made sense. But this is the way I really recall them.

I was flying down a long marble staircase. I felt like Cinderella arriving at the ball. There was music, and men and women dressed in white wigs and crinolines. But I looked down, as I flew, and I saw that even though I was fully dressed, my pussy was clearly reflected in the shiny floor, and that everybody could see it. There were gasps all around, and I saw some of the men looking at me very slyly.

Then I was driving a strange car round the neighborhood where I used to live as a child. I haven't been back there since I was ten years old, and this is the first time I can remember dreaming about it. It was evening, and the sun was hidden behind the roofs and the chimney stacks. There were some children playing ball in the street, and I thought, 'I must be careful not to run any of them down. One of them may be me.' Then I saw a naked man with a black fire chief's helmet on, running down the street towards me. I was frightened he was going to attack me, so I put my foot on the accelerator, but my foot went right through the floor of the car on to the road. The man pressed the end of his penis against the car window and was grinning as if he was mad.

I don't recall what happened next, but then I was sitting at home, trying to read a book of extraordinary pictures. The pictures were in full color, and they seemed to move around as if they were alive, so it was impossible to decide what they were. Even the captions underneath them changed, to suit whatever was happening in the picture. There was one picture where a very white girl in black underwear was being nailed to a wooden door. She was shrieking out, and it frightened me. They nailed her arms and her thighs, and then they led a huge bull out of a pen, and encouraged the bull to rape her. I could hear the scraping noise of the bull's front hoofs as it tried to rear up and rape her.

There was something about a pair of 'interesting and beautiful' mules. I think someone said that they gave you a climax if you tried them on and was trying to persuade me to slip my feet into them. I kept saying no. I was only wearing a T-shirt, and I wanted to keep my hand between my legs to stop people staring at my pussy.

The next thing I knew, I was in a crowd. We were all walking the same way down Park Avenue, as if we were on our way to see something special. I thought of asking some of the other people what was going on, but they all seemed very serious and even angry, so I thought I'd better not.

After a few minutes, we arrived in a plaza that I didn't even know existed. Five or six women, all naked, were lying on the ground. I didn't know what was going to happen to them, but I had the feeling they were being punished for something. Some guards in black firemen's helmets appeared, and they were leading a group of men who looked like apes or gorillas. They were long-term prisoners from Sing Sing, someone said. The women had been 'unwieldy', whatever that meant, and the prisoners were going to be allowed to rape them, as a punishment.

I stepped out into the open and tried to stop the ape-men from raping the women. I kept screaming that you couldn't blame women for being unwieldy. It was what women *were*. But one of the ape-men threw me down, tore away my clothes, and forced his great blunt cock into me. I was pleading with people from the crowd to help me, but they just stood there without saying a word.

There was something else in this dream, but I don't remember anymore. I know that I woke up feeling depressed and frightened, but also sexually disturbed again.

May 22: I went back to my favorite masturbation technique of pressing my thighs together, and I also looked at some sexy magazines. *Viva* was one of them although it didn't turn me on. I found all the men so faggy.

Nice romantic dream. I was being carried along through a forest by a tall and handsome prince. He wore a crown, and rich blue velvet robes. The forest fringed a wide, clear river, and on the other side of the river there was a glittering city, with all kinds of lights and lanterns and shining spires. The prince and I were riding a huge black horse, but even though we rode for hours, we didn't seem to get very far. That didn't matter. I knew this was a dream, and I wanted it to last forever. I didn't want to wake up.

We spread his cloak down on a patch of damp springy moss. He smiled at me and started to speak in a language I couldn't understand at all. Then, after a few minutes, he said that he was speaking backwards language. I couldn't believe it at first. In the air, in front of my eyes, I saw the words *backwards* and *backwoods*, and I wasn't sure which word he meant. I was frightened that he might be speaking backwards, which reminded me of *The Exorcist*.

But all that fear seemed to fade. We were wrapped up in blankets on a small boat that was sailing across the river. He came close to me, and I could feel his hard cock through the blankets. He said I wasn't to move at all, or the boat would tip over, and we would both be drowned. He pushed his blanket-covered cock right into me, and started making love. The blanket was scratchy and irritating inside me, but somehow that made it all the sexier. There were fires burning on the sides of the river, and I could hear voices singing peculiar songs.

The prince rubbed his cheek against mine and kissed me, and I can remember wondering if he was made of mahogany or marble. Perhaps both. I knew for certain that he couldn't be *real*.

There are nearly forty dreams in this six-month diary, but these few serve to show how much light one dream can shed on another, and how important it is to collect a dream *series*.

After you have written down your dreams like this, it is time to start classifying and analyzing them. Most of the dreams in this girl's diary had some connection with rape, and so she put them in the 'rape' category for the purposes of more detailed interpretation. They had already told her something about herself: that she was struggling to find her own sexual identity as a woman, but felt confused and hampered by the fact that men traditionally take the sexual initiative, regardless of the woman's feelings. What was even more confusing was that, in quite a few cases, she actually enjoyed being taken without her consent. Even worse, in spite of her liberated views, she was still prone to mushy romantic dreams of princes and castles.

To solve the apparent paradoxes in her personality, she had to look very closely at the detailed images of her erotic dreams. Now, how can you tell which images are important and relevant, and which are not? Well, you can't. But a sound first step in finding out is to open your erotic dream diary and work your way through every dream, jotting down all the significant images you come across. For instance, the first dream in this girl's erotic dream diary might yield the following list: railroad car, saucepan lids, itchy seats, man in gray suit, cigar, newspaper, ticket in hatband, Swedes and Italians, perfumes, green tissue, 'a gift for the Wobblies', pink rock candy, snow, seat pattern. Some of these images you might leave out, because if you dreamed the dream yourself, you would know they had no great importance. Similarly, you might include other images that I have omitted. On the whole, it is better to write down too many images than not enough. An image that seems unimportant in one dream may recur over and over again in other dreams, and it will take time for you to understand its significance.

* * *

Apart from trying to interpret individual images, collect all your image lists from every dream in your erotic dream diary, and work out how frequently you dream of each image. Do you dream of catsup bottles four times a month! Do you dream of your father eight times a year? The more figures you collect, the clearer your profile of your personality and your deeper interests in life will become.

This book includes an erotic dream lexicon which may help you to decipher some of the meanings of your dreams. But you should never rely too heavily on any kind of dream dictionary, even if it's as open-ended and creative as this one is. Only your own mind can tell you when an interpretation seems right, or when an interpretation is a possibility, but not quite certain. No two dreams ever have quite the same meaning although women do share similar images and events in their sexual imagination. For instance, one New England woman had persistent sexual dreams in which she had intercourse with her husband's German shepherd. Another woman, from Colorado, had dreams in which she arrived home from work to find a big mangy dog lying in her bed, with a huge scarlet erection, lusting to have sex with her. Both dogs represented their husband's sexual desires in different ways. The New England woman was frustrated because her husband was convalescing from an automobile accident, and she wasn't permitted to have intercourse with him. So instead of dreaming about intercourse with him (which she knew was forbidden), she dreamed of having intercourse with his pet dog. The Colorado woman, who had to work very hard all day and arrived home exhausted, saw her husband's sexual demands as bestial and unpleasant. Both women were having sexual dreams about dogs, and in each dream the dog represented almost the same thing. But the meaning of their dreams depended almost entirely on what they themselves felt about the image. And nobody on earth can tell you what you feel about anything except you.

It is more likely that your dream images will refer to something in your personal memory – something particular and very close to home. It is less likely that they will be generalized symbols. Women do dream about the Terrible Mother and the Ogre Father, not to mention the Huntress and the Black Magician. But they are much more prone to dreams about the man who fills up their car or their cousin Belinda-Jane or Walter Cronkite.

Take the pieces of the jigsaw of your erotic dreams, and scrutinize each piece closely. Put each piece through four levels of questioning. Don't rush the process. If you think hard enough and long enough, you may come up with an answer that you know, deep inside you, is exactly right. Don't be disappointed if that doesn't happen too often, though. Most of the time you'll be interpreting your dreams and saying: 'Well, this dream is *possibly* saying this, and this other dream is *possibly* saying that . . .' It's only when you've collected enough dreams that you'll be able to add up the *possiblys* and say that they look very much like a certainty.

These are the four stages of scrutiny that every dream image should go through:

● Is the image a literal image? Is it just what it seems to be and nothing more? If it's a key, is it nothing more than a key? If it seems to represent more, go on to stage two.

● Do you know what the image means to you? If it's a key, does it unlock a particular door? Do you know why you've dreamed about this particular image – or can you come up with a close guess? If you're not sure, go on to stage three.

● If you check the image in the erotic dream lexicon, does the meaning given there begin to strike a chord? Does it remind you of some idea or some feeling — no matter how vague — that you've had in the past, or you're having now? If not, go on to stage four.

● Is the meaning of the image completely obscure? If it is, make a note of it and put it on a page for 'unknowns' at the back of your erotic dream diary. Don't forget it or ignore it. There may well come a time when you can turn back to it and understand what it says.

When you have a particularly long or vivid dream, or a dream that seems to hold some special significance for you, it's worth making the effort to visualize it in pictures or photographs. A whole dream is a difficult thing to draw, because you often find that you've forgotten backgrounds and locales. But you will sometimes be able to remember a particular detail — a face, a strange shape or symbol, an unusual artifact like a knife or a belt-buckle. Make a sketch of it when you first jot down your dream. It doesn't matter if you can't draw very well. The important thing is to capture your dream memory down on paper so that you can visually compare it with waking life. Your drawing may also help other people to come up with suggestions. When you describe a car or a bunch of flowers in words alone, your analyst or friend can only imagine the cars or flowers that he knows. He may, therefore, miss some important points about your car or your flowers, which you saw clearly in your mind's eye but he couldn't.

Some women find it helpful to make dream collages. They look through magazines or newspapers until they find photographs of things that remind them of their dreams and assemble the pictures together to form an entire erotic dream landscape. This technique is particularly helpful with persistent dreams.

Always be ready to revise your opinion about your erotic dreams, even when you think you've come up with a satisfactory interpretation. When you have a complete erotic dream diary, you'll be able to turn back and re-read some of your past dreams with increasing insight and experience. A dream that once seemed like an innocent sexual romp may turn out to have much deeper implications altogether. Just as you're able to look back on your past thoughts and actions in waking life with the benefit of maturity and hindsight, you'll be able to reconsider your dreaming life as well. A 25-year-old Cincinnati woman says:

I used to have dreams in which I did a blatant striptease in front of everybody in my whole high school class. At the time, when I had the dreams, I used to think they were nothing more than dreams of showing off. But they were telling me much more about myself than that. There was a whole lot of applause in the dreams, and everyone was telling me how great I was. It took me years of experience and a marriage that nearly broke up before I understood what those dreams were about. They were pointing out my lack of confidence in myself and the fact that I needed constant approval to function as a sexual person. If my husband didn't make every single move and constantly reassure me that I was doing all right, I used to freeze up. I thought I was going to be America's Number One Frigid Wife. It was only because he had enough patience to give me the self-confidence I needed that I got everything together. It took three or four years. But the whole thing shows to me how clearly a dream can tell you something, even before you consciously know it yourself – if you understand what I mean.

To get the best out of your erotic dreams, you have to be asking yourself questions about them over and over again. Take the striptease dream we've just heard about. The woman should have asked herself: Why am I dreaming about taking my clothes off in front of my classmates? Am I enjoying it? Are they enjoying it? Why are they clapping?

The way you answer those questions is important, too. You have to remember that *other people only do things in your dreams because your mind is making them*. So if this woman's classmates were clapping when she did a strip-tease, it was because she wanted to think about people applauding her. It didn't mean for a moment that people really did applaud her. This is a mistake in interpretation that a lot of people make, even though it's such a simple error. But you can see that, for this woman, it meant the difference between an interpretation which made her think everyone approved and applauded her and an interpretation which showed how much she was seeking sexual reassurance.

Take a dream in which your boss fires you. The boss in your dream is not a self-motivating character, able to do things that upset you, against your will. He is only a puppet in the theater of your mind. You are probably making him fire you in your dream because you want to relieve some unpleasant tension you've been feeling at work. Everything that happens in your dreams stems from you. Even 'discoveries' about people and situations you didn't think you knew about.

Your dream is a function of your imagination. If you're hurt in your dream or aroused or frightened, it's because your mind is making it all happen. But that, of course, is why dreams are so interesting. They are your internal reaction to the events of the world around you. They are a diary in themselves, and that's why it's worth noting them down whenever you can remember them.

Now you know how to collect and classify your erotic dreams, let's run through some real-life dream samples and see how they were interpreted in detail.

4

Ten Erotic Dreams Interpreted

There's a temptation, when you first discover the world of erotic dreams, to expect too much of them. Full of enthusiasm, you write down all your nocturnal adventures and try to work out what they mean. But after the first three or four you begin to find out that dream interpretation isn't as easy as it seems. Your sexual dreams are so crowded with oddities and inexplicable images that you get discouraged.

That's the moment when you should try all the harder to break through the meaning of your dreams. Good dream interpretation is as much a matter of experience as anything else. And you'll never acquire the experience if you give up before you've tried to interpret at least twenty or twenty-five detailed erotic escapades. A girl once told me that she'd tried to analyze her own sexual dreams, but had never managed to get anyplace with them. It turned out that she'd only tried to interpret four, and one of those was about as sexy as a winter Sunday on Coney Island.

If you have trouble interpreting the first few dreams in your erotic dream diary, don't despair. The more dreams you note down the easier it will be to understand what they mean. Just leave the dreams you can't comprehend and come back to them later. And, as I said before, don't ever be afraid to have second thoughts about a dream's meaning.

To give you some ideas about how to tackle your own dream interpretation, I've chosen ten long sexual dreams from women of different ages, classes, and types, and with the women's own help and suggestions I tried to clarify their meanings. I can't guarantee that every interpretation is precisely correct, because in the world of dreams there is no such concept as 'precisely correct'. All I can say is that each of the women agreed that the interpretations had relevance to their own sexual lives, and that they had learned something about their own erotic personality from them.

To broaden the scope of these interpretations even further, I have chosen erotic dreams of the ten most common types. So if you're prone to dreams about celebrities or pregnancy or lesbianism or rape, you'll be able to get some basic idea of how to start analyzing them.

You'll have to bear in mind that these are only individual dreams, taken out of context of dream series, and that their value is limited because of that. I'd love to show you a whole dream series interpreted, but it would take a book five times the length of this one.

Although your erotic dreams are much more complex than puzzles or coded messages, it's best for the purposes of interpretation to treat them as if they're some kind of conundrum. Professor Calvin Hall goes as far as suggesting that you break your dreams down into lists of objects, emotions and environments. But while this may be useful for his purposes, it seems to me that if you break down the pieces of your dreams too far, you'll end up with nothing more than a handful of meaningless bits. You might dream about automobiles seventeen times and tigers eight times – but how do you know that the automobiles weren't really tigers in some dreams, or that both of them sometimes meant something totally different? One controlled leap of the imagination is often worth more than any amount of painstaking classification.

Before we get into some practical interpretation, there is one other point I want to make. Because of Freud's ideas about dream analysis, and the way in which they have been popularized, many people believe, as he did, that everything you dream about has its roots in some objective event in your past. In other words, if you dream about your brother forcing his penis into your mouth, then the dream is connected to a time when your brother tried to make you eat a stick of rock candy and the fantasies you had about it at the time.

The trouble with this kind of reductive analysis is that it always makes you look deeper than the manifest contents of the dream, always searching for some real event at the core of your flights of fancy. If you insist on doing this, you will never touch bottom. Freud believed that dreams could have several meanings going back and back into your past on different layers of consciousness. Your first interpretation didn't make sense? Then it must have another meaning hidden inside it.

The fruitlessness of this kind of dream interpretation has become pretty clear to most modern-day analysts. It plunges you into a hall of mirrors where anything can mean anything at all or even the opposite, and that doesn't get you any place worth going to at all. Dreams are provoked by all kinds of subjective impulses – not just childhood events – and to try and relate every dream to an actual happening can lead to staggering inaccuracies of interpretation.

As Jung said: 'It is true that there are dreams which embody suppressed fears and wishes, but what *is* there which the dream cannot on occasion embody? Dreams may give expression to ineluctable truths, to philosophical pronouncements, illusions, wild fantasies, anticipations, irrational experiences, even telepathic visions, and heaven knows what besides.'

So, when you start interpreting your own dreams, don't try to reduce your visions of extraordinary sexual activities to everyday banalities. What you dream about may well relate to your everyday sexual life, but if there is inspiration and creativity in your dream – or even if there's fear and panic – don't try and turn it all into Kraft cheese slices. To give you an example, a woman friend of mine dreamed she was Empress of India, and that she was able to command men to make love to her and tell them exactly what to do and how to do it, which gave both the men and her a radiant sense of sexual joy. She ventured the interpretation that this dream referred to a time when her husband had suggested they go to a wife-swapping party. How much can any woman underestimate herself? She was really dreaming about her own sexual abilities, which far outstripped those of her husband, and how she could find sexual and spiritual ecstasy through doing sex her way.

Don't forget, then. When you're interpreting your erotic dreams, don't make the mistake that too many men have throughout the centuries. Don't place too low a value on your sexual imagination and your sexual powers.

Let's start with a rape dream from a 30-year-old Los Angeles beauty consultant and see how we get along with that:

I dream that I'm sitting in a sleazy bar in New York, which is where I originally came from. The bar seats are sticky plastic, the bar itself is greasy and covered in spilled drinks. There's filthy cigarette ash all over the place. Along the bar, on either side of me, real sleazo people are sitting. A guy with a greasy pompadour. A woman with a blotchy red mouth and a cigarette covered in lipstick. A fat bartender. I'm drinking out of a murky glass, some clear liquid that tastes like aniseed. There's a mirror behind the bar, but I try not to look at it. I don't want to see myself sitting in this terrible joint.

All of a sudden, the guy with the pompadour comes over towards me. He's the last guy I want to talk to, because I'm frightened of him. He has cheeks smothered in acne spots and tiny mean blue eyes. He says, 'Do you follow the . . .' and kind of nods his head towards the bar. I don't know what he's trying to say. I shake my head, and that seems to make him angry. He opens a dirty handkerchief, and out roll six or seven of those little pink plastic elephants – the ones that you freeze and drop into people's drinks.

I get frightened and try to leave my stool, but the guy with the pompadour snatches my wrist and presses it against the bar with a set of false teeth. They really hurt. It's like someone biting me. I scream, but I can't get any sound to come out of my mouth. People keep saying things to me. The woman with the red lipstick leans over and says something. But they never seem to finish their sentences. She says: 'Can you think of the . . .' and another man says: 'Yes, do you know the . . .' and they never say what.

The guy with the pompadour pushes me face-first on the counter. I'm still sitting on the stool, but he holds me down like that, with my face against the counter. Then he takes out a switchblade and slits my jeans right up the back, so my bare bottom kind of bursts out of them. Then he cuts open his own greasy jeans, and his dirty cock pokes out. It looks as though he hasn't washed his cock in six months, and I can smell it. Rancid, you know.

He leans over me, and I'm terrified in case he touches my face with his horrible white-headed spots. He grips on to my shoulders, and his hands are like claws. The nails are crescents of black dirt. He starts to pant, and then he clings to my back, and pushes his cock into my pussy from behind, that disgusting cock, and I can actually feel it sliding up inside me.

He starts to have me away, this awful man, and there's nothing I can do to stop him. He keeps whispering threats at me, like he's going to slice my face to pieces, or he's going to cut my back to ribbons, and the more disgusting things he says, the more excited he gets. Nobody in the whole goddam bar does anything to help me. They just watch while this guy rapes me, and carry on smoking and drinking. I feel like dying. I feel so used. But there's something erotic about having to submit to this filthy creature, something I can't put my finger on. I lie there with my face against the counter, and I begin to pray that I won't have an orgasm. I mustn't. If I have an orgasm, I'll have given in to him. It will show that he excites me. I mustn't show that. His oily cock going in and out of me. My clean deodorized pussy and his stinking cock. And then he does more than come. He comes inside me, and he pisses inside me as well, so that his hot piss floods me out and pours out of my pussy all down my legs.

The trouble is, I have an orgasm. I'd do anything in the whole world not to have one, but I do. I weep and I cry that I don't want to have one, but I do. I hear someone dropping ice into a glass, and I know that some kind gentleman is pouring me a martini. The only thing I can think is 'How boring . . .'

You have to know something about this lady before you can understand what her dream is all about. She's 30, as we've seen, and she's a beauty consultant. She's blonde, always immaculately groomed, and she's married to an insurance executive called Gordon. Gordon is as smart and groomed as she is, and together they live in a palatial apartment in an expensive LA suburb. They've been married for six years, and there are no children.

The lady was able to interpret the main theme of the dream herself. She knew it was provoked by the frustrations she felt in her job and in her married life. Together, she and Gordon had built up an existence that was glossy and expensive but had about as much reality and earthiness in it as a TV show. 'Gordon's values were all TV values,' she said. 'I think he only fell for me in the first place because I was always so well groomed – not a hair out of place, not a chipped nail.'

Her erotic dream was creating an exaggerated situation 'of real life', which she felt she had left behind in New York City. Dirt, ugliness, and alcoholism. But at least it was something she could respond to with real emotion – fear and eventually lust. At least it wasn't plastic and sanitized like her life in LA.

The people in the dream played a double role. They represented stock sleazo characters, but they were also reminding her of the stock characters in her Los Angeles cocktail-party life. That's why they never finished anything they were saying. She had never felt that her LA friends had anything interesting to say, and so she never really listened.

The man who raped her, with his greasy hair and his spots, was an embodiment of everything that Gordon would never be. She noticed the cosmetic details like acne and dirty nails because her career revolves around them. Gordon would never leave his private parts unwashed for six hours, let alone six months. She noticed the animal smell of this man, and it stimulated her. In real life she would detest a man like this, but in the dream he represented everything that her sex life didn't have – aggression, domination, earthiness, lust. She didn't want Gordon to become a Hell's Angel, but she did want him to stop being so hygienic.

The pink elephants, which she couldn't quite understand at first, were a dream joke. They were reminding her of the tackiness of her social life.

The mirror which she didn't want to look at was making a more serious point. It was trying to show her herself as she really was – lusty and vulgar. But she turned away because she didn't want to admit it.

There was some masochistic fear in the rape scene itself when the pompadoured rapist threatened her with injury. Fear and sexual stimulation are very closely linked in the effect they have on your autonomic nervous system – the system that controls your breathing and your blood pressure and digestion. That's why some people get kicks out of dangerous sports and perilous situations.

When the rapist urinated into her, he was using her as nothing but a receptacle for his own filth. But it was that feeling of being used that brought her – albeit unwillingly – to her final climax. She wanted a man to treat her roughly for a change. She wanted to feel exaggeratedly feminine. She didn't want a man who was all clean fingernails and immaculate BVDs – the kind of man who blathered about 'mutual respect' and asked her if she felt like a cuddle tonight.

The final moment, when someone poured her a martini, was the most telling moment of all. It didn't actually occur in this dream, but at the end of a similar rape dream she had two weeks later. I attached it to the end of this dream, which was clearer than the later dream because it made a typical dream joke point. The beauty consultant herself was able to follow the joke and decipher it. Martini = gin = Gordon's = Gordon. And 'how boring,' she thought.

From this rape dream, we can see again that rape dreams in general have very little to do with real rape (or the male fantasy that every woman in the world is dying to be raped). What this woman was dreaming about was her sexual role vis-a-vis her husband, her femininity, and her sexual identity. She didn't want to have a man who treated her as a germ-free kewpie doll. She wanted to behave like a lustful woman and have her husband treat her like that, too. She also wanted an out from the plastic-molded society she was living in.

This is necessarily a very concise interpretation, and there were other relevant meanings in the aniseed drink, the false teeth, and the conversation. The woman herself could understand what they were, but it would take a chapter-and-a-half to explain them to anyone else. On the whole the meanings were very clear, and there wasn't much deep digging to be done.

Let's take a look now at a marriage-and-home dream. These are often much more obscure than rape dreams because they deal with the raw nerves of married life and personal security. This dream comes from a 25-year-old housewife from Trenton, New Jersey:

I had this dream I was waiting for the plumbers to come and fix the shower. I was standing by the window and looking down the street. I wanted the plumbers to come real bad. I felt itchy, like I was bursting to go to the toilet. But it wasn't like that. It was more like frustrated, when you're frustrated. I was wearing my blue baby-doll nightie, but without the panties. Allen, that's my husband, he brought it back from Boston once. I was naked. Underneath the baby-doll, I was naked.

Then the plumbers were there. I don't know how they got in. I didn't hear them knock on the door. There was two of them. They were wearing blue coveralls. One of them was blond and the other was kind of brown-haired. They came over and they started to take off their coveralls. They didn't say nothing. They smiled, and I smiled back. I knew they was friends.

I took them upstairs, into the bedroom. I looked at the bed and I thought about Allen. I didn't want to have sex with the plumbers on the bed I shared with Allen. I said to the plumbers: 'We can't go paddling in here.' They seemed to understand. We went into the spare room, and the plumbers took their shirts off. They was naked, and I laid down on the bed, and they laid down beside me. The naked plumbers, one each side. Then one got on top of me, and the other held his prick, so that his prick would go inside me all right. And his prick went right in, and the plumber who was fucking me said: 'This is my pipe. Ain't that a great laugh?' Those were his actual words, as I remember them.

I was just fucking the plumbers, and we was going up and down on the bed like it was a boat or something, and I was having a good time. I wanted to do this, I was thinking. I love Allen, but I wanted to do this. To fuck other men. Then I heard the door downstairs, and I knew it was Allen come home, I had to call out, 'Hello, Allen.' He came upstairs and he knocked on the spare room door. We all kept quiet. He knocked again, and I was frightened.

The plumbers managed to climb out of the window, and get away. I opened the door and Allen was standing there. He looked funny. He was pale, and he was wearing a purple-colored suit. I asked him if he was dead, and he said no he wasn't, he was fine. He said he wanted to talk to me about something. I said no, let's fuck. Because I was all worked up by those plumbers, and I hadn't come off, and I wanted to fuck real bad. He said no, he didn't want to fuck. I reached inside his pants, and pulled his prick, but all I could feel in there was a woman's cunt. I asked him if he was a woman, and he shook his head. I said I know you're a woman. That's why you don't love me. You can't love me. But I said — even if we're both women, I can still love you. We can still make love, and fuck. Other women do it.

He said no, and started to slide backwards down the stairs. I knew he was going out of my life. I stood at the top of the stairs and opened my legs. I held open my cunt for him. He slid up and down the stairs, standing upright, and each time he came to the top of the stairs, his cock went into my cunt. I wanted to hug and hold him, but he kept sliding away down the stairs. In the end, he got smaller and smaller, like a tiny doll, and ran away into the sitting room. I shouted out: 'Wait! I can make you bigger, you know!' but he was gone.

This dream — one of a long series — is an illuminating portrait of this woman's marriage, home, and frustrated sexual situation. As a girl, she was ignored by her father, who undereducated her so that the potential of her mind and talents had never been fully exploited. Apart from stultifying her intellect, this chauvinistic upbringing had also confused her sexually because she was unable to express her considerable warmth and passion, and she was also reluctant to show her emotional attachment for any man who was going to treat her like her father did.

The man she married — Allen — was not really capable of giving her the kind of life she desperately needed. She had to have nourishment for her mind, erotic stimulation for her body and emotions, and an opportunity, however belated, to realize herself and her abilities. Instead, Allen's idea of being passionate was to buy her a baby-doll nightdress.

At first glance, it seemed that she was feeling sexually frustrated, and she was waiting for the arrival of some fantasy handymen who could satisfy her needs with some extramarital hanky-panky. But the plumbers had more to their characters than appeared at first sight. They were not just walking dildoes. I encouraged this woman to think very hard about them, and she began to come up with some random associations that threw some interesting light on their role in her dreams.

She thought of them as *plummers* rather than *plumbers*. Connected with plums rather than sanitary fittings. They carried bags, she remembered, that may have been full of plums. Plums didn't evoke any childhood memories or recent waking experiences, but they did seem to stir something inside her mind – some whisper of relevance and meaning. We tried all kinds of ways to stir that meaning up. Ancient dream books told her that plums signified radical changes in circumstances to come. Modern dream books told her that plums were related to breasts. But she finally tracked the meaning down through the use of Webster's New World Dictionary. Plum, it says, is 'something desirable' – and that definition reminded her of a friend, who had told her two or three years before that she had landed a plum job and was completely satisfied and fulfilled. She could even remember the pang of jealousy she had felt when her friend told her that – a pang she had painstakingly buried in her subconscious. She was so sure that 'the plummers' were poignant reminders of that incident that I believe we have to take that as the definitive interpretation of her dream. She was dreaming that, if she was visited by the chance to fulfill her mind, she would also be able to fulfill her body. The whole dream, in fact, is a rather damning indictment of the way in which a father's prejudices and a husband's inadequacies can completely sterilize a woman's latent talent – both intellectual and sexual.

She was still quite loyal to her husband in the dream – something which doesn't often happen. Usually, people dream of adultery without the slightest qualm. The fact that she shied away from having intercourse with two strange men on her marriage bed indicated that her feelings of wifely devotion were still very binding. 'Paddling' was an interesting word. She guessed herself that it could have indicated her feeling that she was dipping a toe into new shallows of sexual experience.

The reference to the plumber's 'pipe' may have been nothing more than a facile dream joke. Freud would have connected pipes with penises, after all. But I advised the woman to reserve judgement on that image. Pipes are phallic, but they are also hollow. Particularly since there was later comment about her husband having a vagina, the pipe may have had some bisexual connotations.

Her marriage vows got the better of her sense of adventure, and her husband arrived home to break up the party. Wearing, you'll notice a purple or plum-colored suit. Could she have been thinking that he had a plum job? Or that he himself was a plum possession? She decided that the answer was most probably the former. She was envious of his job, his career satisfaction, and the fact that he could get out to meet fresh people and friends. But how inadequate he turned out to be! Instead of a penis, he had a woman's vagina, and even when he did manage to make love to her, he dwindled away to nothing. When he was faced with her self-realization, he seemed hopelessly lacking in presence and sexuality. The dream was telling her the truth about her feelings for him.

But it was a hopeful dream. As we've seen, her devotion to her husband was very strong, and even though he was seen in her dream for what he really was – tiny and inadequate – she still loved him enough to offer him some help. The personality lesson that this woman learned from her dreams was that she needed to push herself more. She needed to make her husband understand that she was a person with feelings, passion, and brains – not just a blow-up housewife doll in a shortie nightdress. She had to push it under his nose, rant and rave about it until it sank into his skull that he wasn't married to an undemanding moron. Men blame women for being stupid, but the dumb blond is a completely male fantasy, and men create the kind of social situation in which women like that are considered desirable.

Using the lessons she learned from her erotic dreams, this woman could improve the quality of her life and her sexual relationship with her husband. Both she and her husband would increase in humanity and stature because of it – 'I can make you bigger, you know!'

There was a hint of bisexuality in this dream – even lesbianism. This may have been nothing more than idle sexual curiosity surfacing in her sleeping mind. More likely it was a fairly accurate portrait of her own sexual predilections. All of us have some homosexual ingredient in our erotic makeup, and hers was a little more blatant than most. Lesbianism is not uncommon in the sexual dreams of women who have been badly let down or disappointed by men. With the plain logic of dreams, sexual relationships with other women seem to be less complicated than sexual relationships with men.

Let's go on now to celebrity dreams. As we saw earlier on, these are not necessarily dreams about sex with famous people, but about particular characteristics that you associate with those famous people. This is the dream of a 29-year-old married teacher from Chicago, Illinois:

I know there was an interesting beginning to this dream, but I forgot it as soon as I woke up. I was walking through someone's garden on a hot day in summer. It was a truly beautiful garden – very formal and ornamental, with fountains and flowers and birds. I felt at peace. I was wearing a floor-length white dress with a deep decollete and a pearl-and-diamond crucifix around my neck on a silver chain. On my feet I was wearing little white dancing slippers.

As I was walking along a path between two tall hedges, I saw a man in the distance – just glimpsed him. He had his head bent and he seemed very thoughtful. I found I could glide along the pathways very smoothly and quickly, without even touching the gravel. Bluebirds were soaring all around me and holding the ribbons of my dress in their beaks.

When I arrived at the end of the path, I saw the man disappearing across a meadow, and I decided to chase after him. There was a dark clump of trees in the distance, and I knew that if he got there, I would lose him. He walked very quickly, and wouldn't look back. I tried to shout, but he wouldn't answer. I had a whistle, which I tried to blow, but I knew that the end of it was covered in skin from men's cocks, and I didn't feel like putting it in my mouth.

I glided faster and almost caught up with the man as he was walking between two rounded hills. I called again, and he stopped and turned around at last. I recognized who it was the moment he was close. It was James Mason. He looked tired, and he was carrying a basket with all his groceries in it.

'James,' I said. 'Don't go so fast.' He didn't seem very pleased to see me. I don't know why. I said: 'Are those your groceries?' And he said: 'Yes, I'm thinking of making smearcase tonight.' I said: 'Are we still friends?' and he said: 'As far as I know.'

We walked arm in arm through the garden, which wasn't a garden any longer, but a street in Boston. My grandparents live in Boston, and this was close to their neighborhood. I think I asked James Mason if he knew my grandparents. But he was saying something about 'birthday cakes' and looking very anxious.

The whole scene changed again, and we were back at my apartment in the bedroom. The drapes were drawn, and the whole room was dark. James Mason was sitting on the end of the bed. He was naked, apart from his black knee-length socks. I couldn't resist looking down between his legs at his cock. It was soft, and it was resting there like something sleeping. He had gray pubic hair. I asked him if all men went gray between the legs when they got old. He started producing strings of multi-colored flags out of his ears and blowing his nose on them.

I pushed him back on to the bed, and I spread his thighs with the palms of my hands. I held his balls. They still felt soft, and I could feel the actual balls inside the soft skin. They were like slippery eggs in a velvet purse. His cock didn't seem to rise up straight, but I found that if I leaned to one side, and kind of vaulted over his thigh like vaulting a gate, I could get it inside me. Our legs were all tangled up, and it was kind of awkward, but at least I was actually having sexual intercourse with James

Mason. He was so smooth, you know, and suave. A real mature, beautiful lover. He was holding me so close, so strongly, and yet he was speaking all this wonderful poetry into my ear. I don't recall any of it, really, although there was something about 'the love's limbs and the wonderful workhorse.'

He made me feel so womanly, and whenever I opened my lips, showers of little silver bells fell out, and I knew that I was having orgasms. His cock felt 'as big as a telescope' inside me, and I could go up and down on it as hard and as fast as I wanted. But I didn't want to go *too* fast in case it all ended before I'd had a good chance to enjoy myself. I had an incredible feeling that now I'd had sex with James Mason, I'd be able to join the jet-set. The social elite. It seemed like a whole new life was opening up for me.

This woman's dream seemed at first like nothing more than a jokey nocturnal adventure in which she had sex with a famous movie star. She herself declined to take the dream seriously, and said it was 'silly and childish.' She said she wasn't even a particular fan of James Mason.

She was so adamant that the dream meant nothing at all that I almost abandoned any attempt to interpret it. After all, the assistance of the dreamer is essential in analyzing dreams with any success. But it was what she said about her feelings towards James Mason that made me change my mind and try to solve the meaning of her dream. If she wasn't a fan of his, why had she dreamed about him?

If you dream about a celebrity or a movie star, one of the first steps in your interpretation (unless it's already clear why they appeared in your dream) is to study their public image. What kind of parts do they play in movies? What *impression* do they generally make on people – yourself included? Think of James Mason and do a little free association with words: mature, cultured, European, anxious, deliberate, sophisticated, perverse, intellectual. This is the list I made. Then I went back to the woman and asked her to tell me about her husband. The kind of words I got about him were very different. Extrovert, brash, outdoorsy, athletic, gregarious, straight-forward.

So whatever James Mason represented in her dream, he was certainly the polar opposite of her husband. Now this is where we have to be careful not to fall head first into the Freudian trap of supposing that just because she dreamed about a sophisticated man like James Mason, she was wishing that she were married to a man like that rather than her husband.

I'm not dogmatically saying that she wasn't dreaming about that, but we have to keep our minds open until we know all the facts. Much more frequently, when women dream about adulterous sex with celebrities, they are wishing the celebrities' qualities on their husband, rather than fantasizing about having sex with someone different. That may be a reason why women rarely have pangs of guilt when they are sexually unfaithful in dreams – their dream lover is just their husband in a new and improved manifestation.

Gradually, through intensive questioning, the meaning of the dream became clearer. I still can't claim to have solved it beyond dispute – because the woman herself remains unsure of the interpretation – but it was a reasonable working solution which will help her to interpret other dreams of celebrity sex in the future.

The dream began in an ornamental garden. She remembered an earlier 'interesting' beginning, but it was likely that this was the end of a previous dream. Whatever it was, she forgot it beyond recall, and so nothing could be done to salvage it. Because of later images in the dream, there was good reason to suppose that the garden represented the woman's mind as she saw it. Orderly, peaceful, full of flourishing ideas and beauty. She was wearing a virginal white dress, which could be interpreted as symbolic of virginity and purity, but whose innocence was somewhat compromised by a deep-cut neckline. It was more likely that this outfit represented her concept of herself: a physically attractive married woman with clear, unconfused thoughts. Jewels like diamonds and pearls often signify clarity and uncorrupted ideas – the balanced and perfect self – self-confidence, honorable sexuality, and inner wholeness.

In other words, in her dream, this woman saw herself as a self-contained human being of high moral, intellectual, and physical qualities. But something was missing. This Garden of Eden, her mind, was lacking an Adam. There was a beautiful and humorous image of herself in the way she floated to meet her lover with bluebirds holding her ribbons. She was Snow White, from the Disney epic, wishing to herself that 'someday my prince will come.' When she turned her attention to that sequence again, she was able to remember that the bluebirds were cartoon bluebirds. That's how deep American popular culture goes.

She met her man after pursuing him across a strange landscape. I asked this woman to draw the landscape. Two rounded hills, with a clump of trees in the distance. Landscapes sometimes represent the human body, and her drawing made this abundantly clear. The drawing looked exactly like a woman's body from her own point of view, looking down at herself. She was looking for someone to satisfy her body as well as her mind.

There was a sharp little dig at her husband's superjock athleticism in the image of the whistle. Yes, it was a sports whistle. And yes, it probably represented her disinterest in the kind of sexuality that her husband was offering her.

James Mason, when she caught up with him, looked tired. She felt sorry for him. His tiredness gave her a chance to sympathize with him, offer him some warmth. What you need, James Mason, is a woman like me who can do all your marketing for you and your cooking for you and share your bed. The smearcase image was more tricky. Smearcase is Anglicized from the German schmier-kase, or cottage cheese. Her grandparents used to make it, and when she was a child, she used to sit in their Boston kitchen, eating cottage cheese and listening to her grandfather talk about his happy days at Basle University. Smearcase to this woman had strong associations with culture and European attitudes. Complicated stuff, but it seems to fit in with the general theme of the dream.

Why James Mason was worried about birthday cakes we shall never know. Neither shall we ever know why he was pulling flags out of his ears. It reminded the woman of a magician she had once seen, but she could not explain why she dreamed about it in this way. I hazarded a guess that he might have been showing off his intellect by producing multicolored ideas out of his brain – but why blow his nose on them afterwards? I told the woman to make a note of *pennants* and *flags*, to see if she dreamed about them again, in dreams where their meaning was clearer.

After an awkward act of intercourse, in which the woman herself took the initiative, she felt pleased because she was now a member of the jet-set. She felt, in fact, that her talents and her brain were being appreciated for the first time. I found the poem about 'the love's limbs and the wonderful workhorse' quite interesting. It wasn't a quotation from a real poem, so it must have been created by the woman's own dreaming mind. Did it signify anything? She thought about the words for weeks, without success, until her husband came home one evening after a game of squash and told her several times he had had a 'wonderful workout' with his partner Rosslyn. She began to suspect that James Mason's romantic verse was actually a reference to 'Rosslyn and a wonderful workout', although she could never quite be sure.

The only possible hint of guilt or conscience for her extramarital activity came when she showered bells out of her mouth. According to several ancient sources, bells are a warning of misdeeds, although I suspect that these interpretations were meant to refer much more to church bells and alarm bells. More likely, these bells were tinkly joy-bells and were nothing more than a graphic visualization of sexual delight.

So – taken as a whole – what did the dream mean? It showed that the woman felt deep dissatisfaction with her marriage, both on a sexual level and on an intellectual level – particularly on the intellectual level. It showed that she felt the way to greater personal fulfillment was through an older, more sophisticated man. Or perhaps through her husband taking the trouble to understand her needs, and behaving less like an athlete and more like an emotional and sexual partner.

This is a notable example of a dream that needs to be interpreted in the context of a whole series. If the central situation repeats itself, whether it's with her husband or with James Mason or with Peter Falk or with anyone at all, then this interpretation is probably near the truth. But if she dreams about James Mason in completely different contexts, then we're probably talking about a different kettle of fish. Now there's a potent symbol for you.

You can rarely mistake birth-and-pregnancy dreams for something else. Sometimes, they are very obscurely veiled in puns and metaphors. But most of the time they deal with the plain old obstetric facts. Men sometimes dream about birth and pregnancy in a very clouded way, but women are not afraid to face up to the facts of their own sexual functions and their own sexual organs.

From the few samples I have seen, it appears that women

who haven't had children experience dreams about pregnancy that are not noticeably different from women who have. The only clear reason for this seems to be that a woman's internal concept of herself as a producer of children does not alter in any radical way from virginal youth to prolific middle age. Psychologically, there is not a great deal of difference between the little girl who cuddles her dollies and the mature woman who produces living babies. Men often dream of birth as a trauma, with pain and blood and agonies of muscular contraction. Nandor Fodor, in his book *New Approaches to Dream Interpretation*, suggests that we go on dreaming about the shock of our own birth for the rest of our lives, and correlated some dreams with the actual facts of the dreamer's birth as supplied by the dreamer's mother. But even though women do dream of pain and fear in connection with birth and pregnancy, they also have dreams of extraordinary satisfaction and fulfillment.

What particularly interests me about birth-and-pregnancy dreams is that they very often have a prophetic content. Women who have actually given birth don't seem to dream of birth. But women who are pregnant, thinking of becoming pregnant, or even resisting the idea of becoming pregnant can quite often have futuristic dreams about what's going to happen when they produce. Quite frequently it is an understandable anxiety about the unborn baby's health and wholeness that provokes the dream. But the dream that follows, from a 23-year-old laboratory assistant from Cambridge, Massachusetts, is something different:

I dream that I am sitting at home making paper flowers. They are very difficult to make, and I am having a hard time folding up the tissue and sorting out the wire. I prick my fingers several times. Something tells me that I ought to go and look at myself in the mirror. I walk across the room, where there's a full-length glass, and I'm amazed to see that I'm pregnant. I'm wearing a flowery smock, and my stomach is sticking out a mile.

I'm holding a paper flower in my hand, and it begins to talk to me, in a very papery kind of whisper. It says that I'm due to give birth in sixty-six days, and that the child is going to be a boy. When the flower says that, I catch sight of a small naked body walking down the passage just outside the living room door. I open the door, and he runs away. I think it's very inconsiderate of him to have been born already, without even taking the trouble to involve me.

I chase the boy through all the different rooms in my apartment. At last I catch hold of him. He turns around, and he's a fully grown man — still naked, with a very large and very erect penis. I understand somehow that this is my son, and yet not my son. It is a son who wants to father my son. It's all very complicated, but at the time it seems to make some kind of sense.

I am smiling. I am naked as well, and hugely pregnant. My breasts are enormous, like huge melons, and my stomach is tight and hard. I reach forward and grasp this man's penis in my hand. I feel content. There is warm sunlight slanting into the kitchen where we're standing. It shines on the onions hanging by the icebox. It shines on this man's hair and on his skin and makes his pubic hair look like threads of gold. I caress his penis with warmth and love, and each time I stroke it, he sighs and his muscles tighten. Soon he throws back his head and clenches his teeth, and a warm sticky river of sperm flows over my hand.

I cup my hand and there are four or five drops of sperm in it. I look at them closely, and I realize for the first time in my life that if you look hard at a man's sperm, you can see tiny embryos in it. I don't want to waste them, these babies, and anyway I want to show off that I've had them, so I get them to link hands — they're only about an inch long, but they're all perfectly formed — and I put them around my hair like a hairband or a chain of flowers.

Then I feel a real weird feeling, like the whole of my stomach is dropping down an elevator shaft. I walk quickly across the room, and in the corner is a high-backed chair which I know is a 'baby chair'. I remember that it's all covered in brocade, and it has high gold-painted arms and legs. There's a hole in the seat, and I sit over the hole. Then I push and I push, and gradually the baby squeezes out of my vagina, and disappears down the hole in the chair. There's a kind of chute underneath, and the baby reappears, all clean and naked and smiling, out of the front of the chair.

I pick it up. I'm amazed how heavy it is. It's a little boy. I toss him up and down in the air, and he laughs. He's so beautiful I feel like crying. I suck his penis and it makes him laugh even more. It seems really weird now, but at the time it seems like the natural thing to do.

I suddenly remember all the tiny babies in my hair. I reach up and touch them, and there's nothing but a crown of dead cornflowers in my hair. I look at the little boy I already have, and I hold him real close, and I feel so sad for all the babies that never were.

I love this dream. It's the sort of dream that a man could never have. It has totally feminine attitudes toward sex, and even the typical male sex fantasy of 'floods of sperm' is translated into female terms. Men tend to think of their sperm as a sign of their virility and their domination over women. Its qualities of impregnation they prefer not to dwell upon. But a woman can understand the significance of sperm in context. She is the one who brings the sexual act to its ultimate conclusion, by growing the child in her womb and giving birth to it.

Before interpreting this dream, I had to know something about the girl who dreamed it. It was not an easy dream to fathom, and if I hadn't had the girl's fullest cooperation, it would have been impossible. She's single, although she's been going steady with the same man for two years, and she eventually plans to marry. She was impregnated by this man about a year-and-a-half before she had the dream, but the child (a boy) was lost after four months of gestation.

Once we knew about her miscarriage, much of the dream's imagery became clear. The babies who died and who never were have obvious associations with the child she lost. I tend to think that this girl linked flowers very closely with babies, and that the paper flowers she was making at the beginning of the dream could have represented an attempt to produce another baby – a substitute for the lost child. But it was difficult – both emotionally and physically. The word 'prick' appeared very clearly in her mind when she was thinking about making these artificial flowers, and I believe that for once we could safely say that there was a strong double-entendre in her thoughts. Professor Calvin Hall, among others, has noted the appearance of male and female sex organs in dreams under their slang disguises ('tool' and 'pecker' for penis; 'box' and 'pot' for vagina). In this girl's dream, her attempts to make a new baby involved *wire* ('pulling the wire' is slang for male masturbation) and being *pricked* by wire.

Flowers, incidentally, have traditionally close links with the female sex organs, with growth, 'blooming', and reproduction.

The next sequence was more complicated. Out of the corner of her eye, she saw her child already born and already walking around. He was elusive, difficult to catch, and when she did finally corner him in the kitchen, he was a fullgrown man. He was both father and son in the same personification. It reminded me of that paradoxical saying that 'the child is father of the man.'

I don't think there was much doubt that the little boy was a dream image of the son this girl had lost. But his appearance was not morbid, as it might have been in a man's dream. He was, instead, a representative of hope and optimism. 'I felt he was comforting me,' she said later. 'I felt he was telling me not to have any regrets.'

The father/son produced semen which contained tiny babies, and she wreathed these babies in her hair as a memento to all the babies who are never conceived or who die during labor. This girl was brought up a Roman

Catholic, and although she had lapsed, she still believed in the Catholic view of contraception.

But she really was pregnant in the dream, and she began to feel labor pains coming on. I liked the 'baby chair', which was simply a surrealistic interpretation of birth. She produced her boy, and he was alive. But the price for the birth of that particular child was the nonexistence of all the other children who might have been conceived by the same ejaculation of semen.

This birth-and-pregnancy dream is not wishful thinking, and it's not a mystic prophecy. It's a dreaming drama in which the girl is coming to terms with the idea that not all sperms and eggs can come together to form babies, and that not all babies, once conceived, can survive. But the babies who do survive, in some measure, fulfill the lost promise of those who don't. She lost one child – but another one, when it comes, will give her the maternal satisfaction she wants.

She was slightly worried about the image of sucking her own baby's penis, but this was not sexually significant. Papuan mothers used to suck their babies' penises to soothe them, and it seems to me to be far more of a mothering act than a sexual one.

We've already seen that dreams of public nudity can have many layers of meaning, and many different shades of interpretation. Quite often, they can tell you just what you feel about yourself physically, and the sexual dream that follows, from a 28-year-old housewife in St Louis, Missouri, is a prime example:

I'm driving my husband's station wagon through downtown St Louis, and the problem is that I'm completely naked. I'm wearing my pearl necklace and my high-heeled shoes, but that's all. I say it's a problem, but it doesn't feel like a problem. My hair's coiffured real beautiful, and my nails are manicured, and I feel real sexy and nice. I have a good figure, you know, and a good bust, and I know that people are looking at me driving this car and I'm pleased.

Suddenly that wagon gets squeezed between traffic on both sides, and I'm worried that I've scraped it. I know Jack will be real mad at me if I've damaged it. I climb out and some cop comes over and looks me up and down. Instead of pulling out his notebook, he pulls out his dingus and starts to beat off. I look around, and every car in the whole street has stopped, and every driver has climbed out of his car and is standing there with his cock out, beating off. I start to walk up and down the street like a burlesque stripper, waving my butt around and bouncing my tits. It feels so great to be nude and free in the street – and all these guys beating off, just because of me.

But then, in the distance, down the end of the street, I can see my husband coming. I know he's going to be angry because I've been showing myself off in front of all these strange guys. So I start to run away. I know that I'll have to hide. And the trouble is, people are starting to look hostile because I'm naked. Suddenly, it just isn't sexy any longer. It's embarrassing.

I run into a house, and there are four or five people there that I know. They're playing Monopoly and doing jigsaws, and one of them's playing the piano, but they don't seem to want to notice me at all. I feel they're trying to act superior, because I'm nude and they're not.

I run into another room and I find myself in the middle of a cocktail party. Everyone's talking and laughing, but they soon quiet down when they notice me. I'm real embarrassed, but I know that the men are attracted to me, and they start coming towards me. I can even hear them panting. I sing and swing my pearls around, and I act just like a stripper again, waving my breasts in front of their noses, and groping them between the legs.

The situation kind of changes again. This time – it might be a different dream, but I'm still naked – I'm lying flat on my back on a beach. I know where it is. It's Florida, where we went for our vacation last year. But Jack isn't with me. I'm on my own. I'm lying there in the sand, with my arms and my legs spread wide, naked.

I look up. It's difficult to see, because of the sun, you understand, glaring into my eyes. I look up and there are crowds of people standing around, staring at me. They're talking and chattering, and someone is saying something quite close to me that I can hear over and over again. They're saying something like, 'She's beautiful, she's very attractive, but she's a whore.' In the dream, the word 'whore' sounds like a compliment. I feel like a whore. I feel whorish. After all, I have a good body to offer, why not offer it? If men want to buy, I'm in the market.

But I can see Jack's face again, at the back of the crowd. He's seen me and he's angry again. In fact, he's furious. He starts to push and shove through the crowd, trying to get through to me. I stand up and start to run. The whole crowd chases me. I'm stark naked, running down the road, with a whole bunch of men and women after me, and everyone's lusting after me, you know. They want to rape me.

I run down a kind of alleyway. It's knee-deep in garbage. I reach a fence at the end of the alleyway, and I'm just climbing up it when a man seizes me from behind. I drop back down, and I fall straight on to his big hard dingus. It takes my breath away. It's like jumping into a cold swim-pool on a warm day.

I reach behind me, and I realize that the man who's raping me is Jack, my own husband. He turns around to face the whole crowd, and he says: 'I'm going to fuck her in front of you, just to prove that she's mine.' I'm still standing with my back to him, and his dingus is still buried deep between my legs. He lifts my legs clear of the ground, so that I'm sitting on his dingus with my feet waving in the air, and he starts to fuck me with big long thrusts. There's about forty or fifty people just standing there watching while his enormous thing goes in and out of my body. I love it and I hate it, both at once. I stretch my arms up in the air and I start to crow like a goddam rooster. I make so much noise that I wake myself up.

Although this dream had episodes that reminded me of *The Happy Hooker Meets the Keystone Kops*, it was essentially tackling a serious sexual problem. This house-wife was married six years ago, at the age of 22, and a short time after she and her husband were married, it became apparent that he wasn't the free-and-easy type she had originally thought him to be. He was extraordinarily jealous and made a scene if any other men made any sign of recognizing her or smiling at her or even talking to her. Because she loved her husband – and also because she was flattered by his obsessive behavior — she tolerated the claustrophobic existence he built for her. She was never allowed to go out alone, and if she talked to any men at all, she was frequently subjected to a third-degree grilling when she got home.

This dream was the dream of a woman who felt that she had been stifled. She needed to flirt, she needed to talk provocatively to other men, and above all she needed some confirmation that she was still sexually enticing. As another housewife told me: 'George can tell me I'm sexy until he's black in the face, but that doesn't make me feel any sexier. I need some other man to tell me I'm sexy. I won't be unfaithful, but at least I'll know that George isn't just saying it out of loyalty. Christ, I'd hate a man to tell me I was sexy because he was being *loyal*.'

So our housewife from St Louis, her exhibitionistic femininity repressed, had erotic dreams about it. First of all, she was driving her husband's car downtown. She wore pearls and shoes, which showed that she had dressed up this way deliberately. It wasn't a silly dream accident that she was naked: She obviously meant it to be this way. Notice that she didn't feel shy or ashamed or embarrassed. On the contrary, she was flaunting herself. She was involved in a car smash which damaged her husband's car, and that's a situation that could be interpreted as a way of showing her contempt and rejection for him and his possessions. She was *worried* about scraping his car, but not so desperately worried that she spent the rest of the dream fretting about it. No — she was determined to show herself off. She did a burlesque-style strip, complete with bumps and grinds, all the way down the street.

She ran when her husband appeared on the scene. She was enjoying herself — she didn't want to have her fun spoiled by his possessiveness. She hid in a house where people were playing Monopoly and doing jigsaws. Why

Monopoly and jigsaws? She thought back on this scene, which hadn't seemed very important to her at first, and began to ask herself questions about it, Gestalt-style, by taking the part of the people who were playing the games and doing the puzzles. After a while, it appeared that the game of Monopoly was a dream realization of something she had often said to her husband: 'Do you think you've got a *monopoly* on me?' The jigsaw was possibly a way of summing up how she felt about her life: puzzling, incomplete, fragmented, and yet relentlessly following a predetermined shape.

Next – the cocktail party. I have come across several dreams of people appearing nude at parties, and they are mostly accompanied by acute embarrassment. But not this lady. She was confident of her sex appeal – sure of her physical attractiveness. She began to bump and grind again and inflame everyone in sight. Then she was lying nude on a beach, with people admiring her. Even the idea of being considered a whore didn't faze her in the slightest. There is no doubt that she has a pretty unshakable belief in her own erotic magnetism.

But then her husband chased her and actually caught her. He had sex with her in front of a whole crowd of people, telling them unequivocally that she belonged to him. What made this part of the dream so interesting was that she seemed to enjoy being publicly possessed by her husband. If she enjoyed it, did that mean that perhaps she wasn't so anxious about his jealousy as she might have made out?

Well, there was no question that his jealousy was irksome, and that a woman with her sex appeal and self-confidence would have liked a slightly longer chain on her collar. She would have enjoyed flirting with other men and going to parties in daring dresses. But what her husband obviously didn't understand was that she was completely faithful to him. Much of her confidence was actually founded on his jealousy – the security of knowing that if she did ever try to stray away from him, he would show his husbandly teeth in a big way. She felt, rightly or wrongly, that she *belonged* to him, and because she belonged to him and never questioned that she did, she didn't see why it shouldn't be perfectly all right for her to tease other men. After all, she would always come back.

I'm not in favor of husbands and wives feeling that they own each other like Ming vases or Siamese cats. People are not property. But many women are very dependent on their husbands, physically and emotionally, and this woman was one of them. Perhaps she could learn from her dream (and others like it) that it would be worth her while to try a few steps on her own, and force herself to be a little more independent. Unlike the slaves, women can't be released by laws – they can only be released by themselves. All the manhole covers that have been renamed peoplehole covers, all the children's books that show daddy washing the dishes and mommy going out to work, all the burning of bras and the consciousness raising – this is nothing compared to one woman's realization that she can be free of total dependence on her husband and actually doing something about it. Erotic dreams like these can tell a woman what potential for freedom she has in her personality, and how she can use it.

From dreams of public nudity, we turn to dreams of lesbianism. These can be very exotic and mysterious, particularly if you are not overtly homosexual. Erotic dreams become more cloudy and symbolic in almost direct proportion to the embarrassment you feel about their contents in waking life. In other words, you will probably have quite clear and explicit dreams about intercourse, especially with someone to whom you are lawfully married. But your mind will suppress dreams of less savory activities, and wrap them up in riddles. It's hardly surprising. Even when your mind's awake, it has very confused thoughts about homosexuality and other sexual variations.

This is the lesbian dream of a 40-year-old divorcee from Washington, DC:

A woman friend of mine and I were crawling slowly across the floor of a bakery. We were covered in flour. It was all over our faces and in our hair. I knew it was my brother's wedding anniversary the next day, and I was there to bake him some cookies, but because we had to crawl around the floor, it was hard to get anything done.

I was lying under one of the bakery tables, covered in a floury sack, when I saw slim ankles in tall shoes walking across the floor. I looked up, and I saw it was a 'Muffin Girl'. She was wearing a tall white chef's hat and a small white apron, but when she turned around I saw she wasn't wearing anything else. Her bottom was bare and dusted with patches of flour, and it wobbled when she walked. She had small breasts, but the apron barely covered them, and when she leaned forward to roll out the pastry, her bare nipples appeared on either side.

When the Muffin Girl cut the dough, it fell in long strips from the table. I held on to the end of one of the strips to try and pull her towards me. I only wanted to hold her hand. I only wanted her company. But the strips fell away, and coiled up on the floor like fat snakes. She walked my way again, and she was leaning up against the table. I could see her hairy vagina. It was only an inch, two inches away from my nose. I reached out with one floury finger, and I stuck my finger up the hole of her vagina. She didn't even seem to notice. I took my finger out, and I noticed that the juice in her vagina had cleaned the top two joints of my finger pink again, while the rest of it stayed white.

The Muffin Girl and I were going to meet each other after work in a vacant lot. It was evening. I walked past the Washington Monument, and the water was pale blue, the same color as the sky. The date was the Septy-third of August. I felt in my pocketbook for the keys to my apartment, and inside was a pair of spectacles I had never seen before. They had strange lenses, like mother-of-pearl, streaked with rainbow colors. I knew it was dangerous to wear them, and I threw them away on the grass.

I knew before I reached the vacant lot that the Muffin Girl was gone. I started to run. I ran down the street in front of the White House. Then I wasn't in Washington any longer. I was in Mexico, where I went last year on business. I was sitting in my hotel room, sitting on my bed. It was very hot, and the sweat was dropping from my face like globs of honey. I was wearing nothing but a shirt, and I was unbuttoning that so that I could go to bed. The insects outside were very loud.

I heard sheets rustling, like someone asleep in a nearby room. I heard a girl sighing and moaning. I turned around, and there was a girl in my bed. She had a mass of black curls and ringlets, all tied up with ragged red ribbons. She was twisted up in the sheets, and she was openly masturbating. She reached out and took my hand, and pressed it between her thighs, so that I had to masturbate her. I didn't want to at first, but she was very beautiful in a sultry sort of way, and I began to feel aroused.

There was a small black animal sitting between her breasts. At first I thought it was there to soak up the perspiration. But when I tried to touch her breasts, it opened its eyes and bit my hand.

I looked down and the girl had worked her way between my legs, and was licking my vagina with her glistening red tongue. She was very sensual, and she kept caressing and squeezing her own breasts, and pinching her own nipples. There was a record playing, a very scratchy one, that I recognized. It was *L'Arle-sienne* by Bizet. The girl had her face pushed right into the cleft of my bottom, and was making loud sucking noises as she drank the juice out of my vagina. She somehow pushed her head right inside my vagina, and licked me from the inside. I couldn't have an orgasm, no matter how much I tried. In the end, I was so frustrated that I dressed myself and packed my case. The girl held my hand, and trotted after me, down the stairs and into the foyer. She was exquisite to look at – I can remember her face now. I've never seen a girl so wildly lovely in my life. She had olive skin, slanting green eyes, full lips, and this tangle of black curly hair. Her breasts were almost ridiculously big, and yet she carried herself so upright that she managed to look graceful. A slender waist and a high, round bottom. Long legs. I had tears in my eyes because she was so sexy and so beautiful and yet I knew it was all a dream and I wouldn't be allowed to stay with her. She was crying, too. We both knew it was a dream, and we didn't want it to end. But I could feel myself waking up. She said: 'Here,' and she took my hand and placed it on her breast. I could actually feel her nipple in my fingers. I thought if I clung on to it, she would stay real, even after I woke up. When I did wake up, I was clinging on to the corner of the pillow, so tight that the ends of my fingers were white.

This lesbian dream is what we call a 'lucid dream'. Not lucid because its meaning is clear, but because the dreamer was aware during the dream that she was dreaming. There are many fascinating examples of lucid dreams (some of the best of which are included in Celia Green's book *Lucid Dreams*). Psychical researchers suggest that lucid dreams could provide evidence that the spirit leaves the body during sleep, and that they might be useful in discovering more about extrasensory perception. One of the qualities which distinguishes a lucid dream from an ordinary dream is that, once the dreamer is aware that she is dreaming, she can participate in the dream and control its course. Dr F. van Eeden, for instance, in his *Study of Dreams* published in 1913, claimed that he could sing and shout in his dreams at will, and yet his wife confirmed that he had slept soundly and peacefully. I admit that nobody checked her for deafness.

The divorcee who dreamed this dream was an intelligent, attractive, but rather lonely woman. She lived on her own, although her younger sister frequently came to stay with her. She had been married twice, and both times her marriages had ended in divorce. She felt suspicious of men, exploited by them, and extremely unwilling to get involved in another long-term relationship.

This is a very familiar background when we are talking of lesbian dreams. Often, lesbianism seems like a way of finding sexual companionship without the hassles of heterosexual love. We are attracted to members of our own sex more frequently than we realize, and it is only our social conditioning that suppresses our thoughts so effectively. In several ancient cultures, bisexuality was considered to be so normal that it wasn't even interesting, and there is no biological evidence that men and women have radically altered since the days of Virgil. When a woman has rejected the idea of a male partner, temporarily or permanently, she is often surprised to find that girls begin to look highly desirable.

The fallacy, of course, is that homosexual relationships are just as riddled with problems and fraught with anxieties as heterosexual relationships, if not more so. They are always under greater social pressure, and if one of the partners is not genuinely lesbian, the emotional stress can be enormous.

However — back to the dream and its interpretation. It started in a bakery, with the dreamer and a woman friend crawling across the floor. She wanted to bake some cookies for her brother's anniversary. This could have been a simple reminder dream, but dreams of cooking and baking have some connection with making an effort to find out the truth about yourself. You take the raw material of unpleasant facts, and you bake it into something more digestible. I wouldn't normally support a dream-book type interpretation of this kind, but it seemed to the dreamer herself to have some relevance, so I've included it.

Then the fantasy lesbian partner appeared — the 'Muffin Girl'. Again, we had a slang reference to sex. 'Muff' or 'muffin' is a slang term for the female sexual parts. Whether the dreamer consciously knew this or not doesn't particularly matter. The coincidence is too neat to ignore.

The Muffin Girl started to cut up raw pastry (the raw facts of life?), and strips fell under the table where the dreamer was hiding. She tried to use them to pull the Muffin Girl toward her, but they fell on the floor like fat snakes, or flaccid penises. Yes — she agreed they were probably symbolic cocks. The raw facts of her life (the dough) were simply that cocks now seemed repulsive and undesirable.

Dreams sometimes have a penetrating attention to detail that helps you to recall them with much greater ease than normal. The way the dreamer's floury finger was moistened into pinkness by the Muffin Girl's vagina was a classic. I didn't believe there were any special implications in this act. It was a straightforward and explicit sexual experiment. The reason the Muffin Girl didn't respond was because the dreamer was only interested at that moment in her own response to the situation. She was too busy considering how lesbian love would affect her to worry about how it would affect a would-be lover.

After work she made a rendezvous with the girl in Washington. I am not a great subscriber to Freud's phallic symbols, but I had to admit in this dream that the Washington Monument could have had phallic implications. But note that it was a *memorial* to male virility, a reminder of the past, rather than a desirable penis of the future.

I was interested by the dream date – the Septy-third of August. It was a nonsense date, of course, but the woman did half-believe in astrology, and for people who believe in it, it can have significance in their dreams. As an experiment, I checked the visual *Dream Scope* of astrologer Sydney Omarr for the period around August-September (Virgo). There were prophetic indications of new love, a breakaway from past conventions, and a warning of a heart broken by a man. There was also, coincidentally, a pair of spectacles. I am not claiming anything for astrological dream interpretations of this kind, but I am pointing out that it is worth keeping an open mind on anything that can throw light on what you are dreaming about.

The dreamer herself interpreted the spectacles as 'a new way of looking at sex . . . but a warning, too, because they were saying that if I took a rosy, rainbow view of everything, I was going to get hurt.'

She *was* hurt. The Muffin Girl wasn't there when she arrived at their trysting place. But the scene changed, and she was in Mexico with another girl, an exquisitely beautiful Caribbean-type creature who was ready for any kind of lesbian adventure. As far as the dreamer could tell, this girl was a fantasy creation out of her own mind. She had never met a girl like this before, and didn't think that she was generally attracted to half-castes anyway. But it was hard to be too conclusive about this. The image of the girl may have come from some long-forgotten movie or magazine photograph.

The black animal between the girl's breasts was another interesting image. It was rather like a cat, and cats are a familiar ancient symbol of powerful femininity. This femininity was dangerous, though – it bit her. There were plenty of warnings in this dream about the possible dangers of homosexual liaisons.

L'Arlesienne by Bizet was a record which had once belonged to a friend of hers – 'a very tweedy, loud-voiced girl.' She had never openly suspected this friend of lesbianism, but obviously the thought was buried down deep in her unconscious mind, and when she began to dream about lesbian activities herself, it surfaced.

The girl actually tried to push her whole head into the dreamer's vagina. This may have been nothing more than a dream-like exaggeration of lesbian cunnilingus, or it may have had some stronger meaning. It may have meant that the dreamer was trying to hide her homosexual feelings inside herself, or that she was actually attempting to assimilate the girl and thereby acquire her sensuality and her beauty for herself – a kind of vaginal cannibalism.

The dream was ultimately frustrating. Because of her inhibitions, the woman was unable to reach orgasm, and derive the satisfaction from lesbian love that she thought she was going to. What's more — even when the dream entered its lucid stage, and she was actually aware that she was dreaming, the lucidity only served to underline her loneliness and frustration.

From this erotic dream, the woman could learn that she was capable of feeling sexual desire for other women, but that her basic emotional makeup was not equipped to find real satisfaction in lesbianism. After a period of 'convalescence', she would find the fulfillment she needed by forming a new relationship with a man. This was not a wish dream but a *possibility* dream — a dream that considered the possibility of lesbianism and then ruled it out.

Incest dreams always make for tricky interpretation. Because you've known your parents and your brothers and sisters for so long, and because they are who they are, it's impossible for you to have any kind of objectivity about them. Because of this, you have to be prepared to consider several different interpretations on several levels of eroticism. Only a longish series of incest dreams will give you a clear view of which of those interpretations is nearest to the truth.

The main point to bear in mind, though, is that few incest dreams really mean that you want to have intercourse with your father or brother, and so you needn't be worried that there's anything awfully wrong with you. The time to start thinking about it rather hard is when you actually feel attracted to them in waking life. In your erotic dreams, they are probably just taking acting parts. They are convenient male faces that your mind knows well, and so they're ushered in to make up the numbers. Dream casting can sometimes be very amateur and arbitrary. Think of putting on a production of *Hamlet* with the staff of your office, and you'll have a pretty clear idea of what your mind does when it stages one of its little mental dramas. You tend not to dream about people you don't know.

Here's an incest dream from a 21-year-old medical student from Indianapolis:

It's midwinter. The sky is black, and the ground is covered in snow. I'm sitting in the back parlor of my parents' house, looking out at the garden. There are blobs of snow on the fence posts, and there are tracks of birds' feet on the windowledge. There is a radio playing somewhere in the house. For some reason, I feel sad and lonesome.

Upstairs, I can hear someone laughing. I walk upstairs. I want to find out what's going on. I feel left out. I walk from room to room, opening and shutting doors. All the upstairs bedrooms seem to be empty. I walk into my parents' room, and there's my mother's dressing-table with all her bottles of perfume and her powders and her lipsticks. I walk over and look at myself in the dressing-table mirror. It's hard to focus on my own face.

I look around and my brother William is lying in my parents' bed. He's smiling at me. The whole bed is covered in broken toys. I sit down on the bed next to him. He is talking about something, but I can't hear him properly. I wonder if there's something wrong with his voice. I keep asking him to speak up, but it doesn't seem to make any difference.

I notice that he's naked, that he isn't wearing any pajamas in bed. I feel very attracted to him, and I slide my hand under the sheet, and I stroke his thigh. He smiles at me. For some reason, he doesn't want to talk anymore. He leans over and kisses me, and I think that at last he loves me.

I lift up my skirt, and he pushes his hand in between my legs, and into my panties. Before he can do anything, I put my fingers to my lips, and I creep over and lock the bedroom door. Then I go back to the bed, and I pull down my panties at the front so that he can see between my legs. He puts his hand there, and starts to turn me on. He's younger than me, and he doesn't seem very experienced, so I hold his wrist and show him how to turn me on best.

I pull back the sheet. His penis is sticking up between his legs. I push him back on to the pillow, and I sit astride him. We start to make love, and I can't describe the sensation of it. I know that whatever we're doing is wrong, but somehow that makes it all the more exciting. I start to have fantasies of what will happen when my brother comes inside me. My own brother — coming inside me! The whole thought of it makes me feel crazy with sex. You know, really excited.

But he doesn't come. Instead, we're standing outside a bowling center in Indianapolis. We're dressed again although I feel uncomfortable, as though I've put my clothes on in a hurry. We're holding hands. But I'm not sure that William is still interested in me. There are some sexy looking girls of fourteen or fifteen standing around the doorway of the bowling center. They have short skirts and tight sweaters. Some of their skirts are so short you can see that they're not wearing any panties. William says: 'Excuse me one minute,' and he walks over and starts to talk to one of the girls. She's nodding and smiling, and I feel very jealous. Then she puts her back against the wall and lifts up her mini-skirt. I can see the dark hair between her legs. William takes out his penis, and they start to have sex, panting like animals. I can see drops of shining liquid running down the girl's bare legs. I'm so annoyed that I run away.

The next thing I can remember, I'm opening a letter. I'm sitting on a train, and I read the letter on the train. I know that William has left me. I don't know why. I feel very sad. I'm a little surprised to see that it isn't winter anymore. The train is running through a bright painting of a field in Georgia where the tracks cross at right-angles, and I feel sorry for myself, and for my brother, and for everyone in the whole of America.

This girl did not come from a particularly tight-knit family, which made it surprising that she dreamed about her brother so jealously and possessively. Some of the time, he may have appeared as a stock male character, but for most of the dream he was playing himself, which led me to think that this dream could contain some interesting revelations about her sexual attitudes.

She was not a lonely girl. She didn't think that she was sexually inhibited, either. She had had three lovers since the age of seventeen, and at the time she dreamed the dream, she was going steady with the latest of them. She claimed to have been 'quite close' to her brother, but not unnaturally close, and they had never done anything sexual together. He was two years younger than she was, and she didn't feel sexually aroused by him at all.

Then why did she have this dream of incest?

Jung might have suggested that the brother/lover was a dream manifestation of her animus, the male side of her personality, and there was possibly some truth in this. One dream dictionary suggested that to dream of having sex with your own brother is a sign of family security. The family that lays together, stays together. But none of this kind of thinking was really getting us down to the central core of what the dream was all about.

One of the strongest clues was in the obscure sequence toward the end of the dream, in which she saw a field in Georgia where the railroad tracks crossed 'and I feel sorry for myself, and for my brother, and for everyone in the whole of America.' I asked her why she felt sorry for everyone. 'Because,' she said, 'I want to help them all and I could never manage it.' In other words, she had a deep sense of social responsibility – even for people she could never do anything for. This was one of the reasons she had decided to become a medical student. We went through a whole sequence of associations connected with social responsibility, and a phrase that immediately caught her attention was, 'Am I my brother's keeper?' Not long before she had had the dream, a student friend of hers, during a discussion on medical ethics, had asked her: 'Are you your brother's keeper?' and she had answered: 'Yes, I believe I am.'

The railroad tracks that crossed at right-angles reminded her of a painting of early America she had once seen, and in her mind it summed up the spirit of the nation as a whole. There were no people in sight, but the whole of the United States lay where those tracks went west and east and north and south. She felt a duty toward people, and her dream was expressing that duty in a visualization of the concept of being 'my brother's keeper'.

Why the protection of her brother should have taken the form of sexual intercourse instead of, say, wrapping his legs in bandages, is a more difficult question. But she hazarded a guess herself that it was because she had recently undertaken a course on sexually transmitted complaints, and she had been shocked by the extreme youth of some of the patients she had seen. She might have unconsciously identified them with her younger brother, and, in her dream, she might have been trying to protect him in a sexual way. Certainly the later sequence, where she saw him having intercourse with a teenage prostitute, seemed to back this guess up.

The broken toys on the bed were a poignant dream image which expressed, more clearly than any words, the passing of childhood. Her brother was now a sexually aware adolescent. He was naked, and she had sex with him. She was excited by the forbidden aspect of incest, but then most of us are aroused by forbidden activities.

After the prostitute sequence, she realized that she could not accept total responsibility for her brother's sexual welfare. Even though she was jealous, and even though she wanted to protect him, he still wanted to have intercourse with other girls. That was why she found herself on a train, traveling away from him and opening a letter that told her he was gone.

I didn't believe for a moment that this girl felt no sexual feelings for her brother at all. Just because they weren't the same kind of feelings she had for other men, that didn't mean that she was totally neutral toward him. It is rare for women to have dreams of sex with people they regard as sexless; it is far more common to have dreams of sex with people you consciously regard as sexless but unconsciously feel some attraction for.

This woman could learn from her dream that she was trying to carry the responsibility for more sorrow and sadness than she could manage. If she was going to be a successful medic, particularly in the sexual field, she would have to learn to be far more objective about her patients. She could learn, too, that dreams tell you the truth, regardless of what you want to think about yourself. She was sexually interested in her brother (as millions of girls are), and it was nothing to worry about. On the same harmless level, he was probably just as sexually interested in her.

You can see from this interpretation how many levels an incest dream can be working on. The brother is an archetype of all young people; he is himself; and he is also the manifestation of a popular phrase. There just isn't enough space to go into all the other images in the dream — the snow and the music and everything else, but they all work on several different strata. Once you are aware of the main key to the dream, you should be able to analyze most of the possibilities yourself.

From incest, we turn to sadomasochism. Earlier on, when we were discussing the ten most common erotic dreams, I gave a masochistic dream as an example. As a contrast, here is a sadistic dream, from a 35-year-old housewife from San Francisco, California:

I had this dream, but I can't remember all of it. I know it was a long dream. It seemed to go on for hours. There was something about a church, and some sort of religious service, but I don't recall that at all much. I do remember most of the sex bit, though. Some of it was real strange, and even when I woke up I couldn't get it out of my head. What I was doing was, I was holding this man prisoner in my hall closet. Can you imagine that? I don't know what he was doing there, or why I was holding the poor guy prisoner, but there he was, naked as the day he was born, and shut up in my little understairs closet. In this dream, my husband and me, we seemed to go on with our lives in a perfectly ordinary way. But I remember thinking that I wanted my husband to go off to work on time, because then I'd be able to have my fun with this guy in the closet.

So David went to work, that's my husband. Then I went to the closet and opened it, and the guy was sitting there. He looked quite like David himself, except he was younger and better-looking. He was tied up with rope, or maybe electrical wire. I pulled him out, and he had to follow me into the living room. I made him kneel down on the floor, on the rug. I said: 'Now, are you going to be good?' and he said: 'Yes, Mrs P——, I'm going to be real nice.'

I held his chin, and I took a long skewer-stick and I pushed it into his cheek, right through his tongue, and out of the other cheek. He didn't try to struggle or cry out. He just looked at me. It makes me sick to think of it, what I did to that nice young boy. But in the dream I couldn't care less. It was just like sticking a skewer in a piece of meat. Now I knew he couldn't talk, couldn't answer back.

I said: 'Are you going to make love to me? Nod your head if it's yes.' So he nodded his head. I knew I had to hurry, because David was coming home soon. I had the idea he'd forgotten something, and he'd have to come back for it. So I hurried, as much as I could. I went to the dresser and I took down glass jars and drinking glasses, and I smashed them all into pieces, and I made a circle of broken glass on the floor. I made the young man sit on all these broken pieces of glass. He didn't have the skewer in his mouth no more, and he was crying out, because the glass was cutting his ass and his balls.

I took off my skirt and my tights and my briefs, and I carefully let myself down on this man's prick. The more weight I put on top of him, the more it hurt him. The glass cut into him, and he was trying not to cry out, it hurt so much. I bit his face and his ears, and then I bit his nipples. I ran my fingernails down his cheeks until they were red and bloody. I looked between my own legs, and his prick was bloody, and his balls were dripping red. I sat down, with his prick up inside my snatch, right up as far as it would go, and I felt this deep thrill up in my womb. I went up and down on him, fucking him real hard, and even when he had his climax, I couldn't stop, and I made him have another and another.

I knew David was coming home. I think I saw his car outside. I tried to push the young man back into the closet, but he seemed

—

to have blown up like a big balloon, and he wouldn't fit in. I knew the calendar in the kitchen had to be changed before David came back. He mustn't know what day it was. And there was blood on the rug. I was naked, and he'd see all the blood on my legs and my snatch, and he'd be furious. I was trying to wash my snatch in the basin when the doorbell rang, and I knew he was back.

The dreamer herself was able to interpret the main theme of this dream — which just goes to show how vivid and clear most erotic dreams are. It reflected a pressing sexual situation that was affecting her marriage at that time. She and her husband were both Jewish, but while she had had a completely free and liberal upbringing, her husband had been disciplined by his father, a severely Orthodox Jew, and was still living his life on very traditional Jewish lines.

As you can probably guess from the dream itself, the problem was that he refused to have intercourse with his wife on days when she was menstruating. At first, this hadn't bothered her. But the more she thought about it, the more it irritated her, particularly since she and her friends had recently discussed the subject at a *kaffeek-latsch*, and she had discovered that most of her friends' husbands had no objection to menstrual sex at all. David, however, was too dominant a personality for her to be able to sway him against his religious principles. Note that the forgotten part of her dream contained some reference to religious ceremonies, which is a fragment of evidence that religious matters were on her mind.

I was fairly satisfied that the man in the cupboard was David himself. Only *this* young man was a David whom she was able to control and dominate. Notice that the dream doesn't go far away from reality at any point — she dominated him physically, but she never dominated him mentally. Just to make sure that he didn't get his own way, she silenced him with a skewer through his tongue. There were religious undertones in this action, too. In the Far East, during the ceremonies of Thaipusam, religious men push skewers and hooks through their cheeks and tongues as a mark of penitence.

The dreamer broke jars and glasses, and made them into a sadistic seat for her wayward husband. The glassware had been given to her by her husband's mother, and using it in this manner may have had some significance. It was an act of vandalism against his orthodox upbringing.

Then she forced him to do the one thing he wouldn't agree to — have sex in a welter of blood. But this time, there was a dreamlike poetic justice going on — it wasn't *her* blood, it was *his*. She emphasized her physical domination over him by biting him and scratching him.

Suddenly, though, she realized the real David was coming home. The David she couldn't handle. She tried to clear away the evidence of her sadistic feelings, and she even altered the date by changing the calendar in the kitchen. The date, of course, was the time of the month when she had her period.

This dream showed the dreamer that she had hidden sexual strength. She didn't usually use that strength, and she allowed her husband to dominate her — a domestic situation that, for both of them, had become something of a habit. But she did have the power to break free from his orthodox attitudes, even though it probably meant that she would have to be hard, determined, and possibly cruel. She was not by nature a sadist, but the dream suggested that she would have to be if she wanted to tilt the balance of power in her favor. Whether she had the right to ask him to break his religious convictions was one thing; convincing him that he should treat her as a free and equal person — and also as a woman — was another.

After this dream, the woman was worried that she might

be turning into a genuine sadist. She had, after all, enjoyed hurting her husband in her dream. It had given her a sexual thrill. But there was really no need for anxiety. While she might have had some sadistic leanings, it was more likely that she was deriving most of her erotic satisfaction out of setting the sexual pace for a change.

Talking of that, it surprised me how many women's erotic dreams featured sexual acts in which the woman herself was dominant. Our society might have brought us up to believe that the only dignified sexual position is man on top, woman underneath, but it sometimes seems that women prefer to be in charge. It rather knocks the bottom out of the idea that sex is something that men do to women. It certainly reflects the feeling of many wives and girlfriends that their husbands and lovers are not sexually competent enough to consider themselves in charge of all their erotic activities. Men understandably resent being told that they're not making love well enough to satisfy their women, but if their women are continually having dreams about taking the sexual initiative, then the men are probably not the Casanovas they like to believe.

In the following orgasm dream the woman who dreamed it tries to solve her own sexual problem, with very productive results. It comes from a 31-year-old restaurant owner from Chicago, Illinois:

I am sitting in my doctor's waiting room, and I know that the doctor is late. I have gone to see him because I have so much trouble with my sexual orgasm. I am thinking what I ought to say to him. Whether I ought to say: 'Well, it's like this, doctor, I can't come,' or maybe I ought to say: 'I'm having such trouble with climaxes, doctor.' But, as it is, I don't have the chance to say either. A woman in a brown dress and a strange mask on her face comes to the door and says that the doctor won't be able to see me. I try to look in through the eyeholes of her mask, but I can't see anything. It's a frightening mask, like an African tribal mask. I don't want to stay, and I run out into the street.

I know that I have to work out what's wrong with my orgasms. This is very important. Something's wrong, something's missing, and I can't go back to work until I find out what the problem is.

I go to a narrow doorway next to a dingy old bookstore. It's dark inside, and I have to force my way through suffocating black blankets and heavy black velvet drapes, until I'm standing in a red-lit room. A young man, stripped to the waist, comes over and smiles at me. I notice that he's wearing earrings, and each earring is a tiny pink woman in a gold cage. I reach in my purse and pay him a handful of dollar bills. He puts his hand up my dress, seizes my panties so that his hand goes in at one leghole and out of the other, and pulls me along after him.

Lying on a black velvet divan is a very tall, very muscular man. He is handsome and silent, and his whole nude body is gleaming with oil. He looks like Adonis — you know, a real dish. He has no hair on his body at all. He has an amazing cock, the size of my forearm, and balls like shining globes. I'm frightened that he's going to hurt me. But he takes my hand and tugs me towards the divan. I lie back, and I'm tense. Every muscle in my whole body is tense. He climbs on top of me, and starts to kiss me all over. My lips, my hair, my nipples. He keeps telling me to relax. I tell him I can't relax. It's impossible. There's no way I can get my tension to ease off. Well, he says, tense your muscles even more. Make your muscles harder and tighter. So I do that. I squeeze my eyes shut and I make myself rigid. Absolutely rigid. Then he says, let go. Relax. And I relax. I go totally floppy and easy and beautiful.

That's when he gently opens my thighs, and slides that giant-sized cock up into me, and I don't feel tense or worried about it at all. I'm just floating. I hold on to him real gentle and easy, and he almost floats in and out of me. I don't feel his weight. All I feel is his cock, easy and long and lovely. The more the lovely feeling increases, the more relaxed I am, until I know that I'm going to have an orgasm. I'm a little worried in case I lose it, now that I know it's coming, but it has complete control of me, and this gorgeous floating man is fucking me and fucking me and I know he's not about to stop.

Even when the orgasm starts to flow up my legs and all over my body and my brain — even then I don't tense up. It's a beautiful agony that runs up me and then down me again, like water in the bathtub when it pours from one end to the other.

I write out a check to this man, to pay him for what he's done.

Instead of a pen, I have to use the hairy claw of some animal. Nobody seems to notice, and so I guess it's all right. Before I leave, I bend down and lift his big oily cock in my hand, and kiss it.

As far as orgasm dreams go, this one was most interesting. Not the least fascinating part was the sequence where the young man finally taught her to achieve satisfactory climaxes, because this had some resemblance to the eccentric and extraordinary orgasm theories of Dr Wilhelm Reich. Reich who wrote *The Function of the Orgasm* in 1942, claimed that negative energy built up in the body. Regular orgasms were required to discharge it, this energy, and thus ensure continuing mental health. Sometimes, you would have too much tension inside you, and Reich discovered that the way to release this tension was to apply extreme pressure. When the rigidity relaxed, you would have a spasm quite similar to an orgasm.

Reich's theories have some dedicated adherents, including movie stars Jack Nicholson and Dyan Cannon. But the official medical view is against his ideas, and there are many valid criticisms of his fundamental arguments. Nonetheless, the restaurant owner lady who dreamed this dream did come up with an interesting way out of her orgasmic difficulties. Relaxation is a major step in achieving sexual satisfaction. Whether she was dreaming a Reichian dream or not, she was certainly going through an intriguing mental process of sexual self-help.

What else could she learn from interpreting her dream? She learned that she was disillusioned with regular doctors. She was still undergoing a course of treatment from one doctor, and she wasn't consciously aware that she had lost faith in him, but the dream said different. She drew the strange mask that the doctor's assistant had been wearing, and when she had it down on paper, she recognized it for what it was. An African witch-doctor's mask. Her erotic dream was telling her, in sarcastic visual terms, that her doctor was no better than a tribal quack.

So, off she went in search of her own answer. There was a sequence in which she had to force her way through suffocating blankets and drapes. This may have occurred because a blanket had actually fallen over her face while she slept, but if it wasn't caused by that, it bore close resemblances to dreams of birth (or, in this case, re-birth). She might have felt that she was entering a new life.

There was another bitter little dream joke in the young man's earrings. Tiny women in cages, dangling from his ears. 'I knew what that meant,' she said. 'I sometimes feel that men treat me as an ornament, a decorative appendage, and not as a woman at all.'

Nonetheless, she sought sexual therapy from the men in her dream, and was introduced to 'Adonis'. As far as she could remember, this man was nobody she knew. He was an archetypal Greek god character, and a complete fantasy of what a sexually attractive man ought to look like. 'In fact,' she said, 'he was so handsome I didn't even find him particularly exciting.'

But the dream therapist, as he made love to her, was not trying to be a lover or a soulmate or a life partner. He was almost like the surrogate partners that Masters and Johnson used to sort out orgasmic dysfunction in some of their patients. Her mind had only created him as a way of saying *relax when you make love, don't get uptight about your orgasms*.

This was an example of a dream that was trying to solve a sexual problem by presenting new possibilities – untried ideas. After she had dreamed the dream, and interpreted its meaning, the woman tried to relax more during her real-life lovemaking, and she found that it genuinely did help her to have climaxes more often – although not as dramatically as it had done in the dream. Your erotic dreams can point out things about yourself that you haven't consciously noticed or that your waking mind refuses to recognize, and that's where they can help you if you have a sexual hangup.

There was one mystifying little image in this dream – the hairy animal's claw she used to write the check. To help her discover what it could have been, I gave her a list of animals, and told her to pick out one or two creatures that the claw could have possibly belonged to. But she was only halfway through the list when the answer came to her spontaneously. It was a rabbit's foot, a good-luck charm that had been given to her by her first lover, when she was sixteen. He had been a skillful and appreciative bedmate, and she had never had any orgasm trouble with him – not like she had with later boyfriends. This image was a fascinating example of the way in which dreams gather together all kinds of random information that may be relevant to your current problems. In the shorthand of dream language – which is often clearer and more precise than waking language – the rabbit's foot was reminding her of that long-ago relationship when orgasms were actually easy.

As a matter of interest, the woman went to the street where she had dreamed the 'sex therapy' building was. The bookstore was real enough – she had passed it a thousand times. The building next door was a delicatessen, with rows and rows of salamis hanging in the window. If that wasn't another case of blatant phallic symbolism, I don't know what is.

Last, let's take a more detailed look at dreams of female liberation. This dream comes from a 27-year-old swimming instructor from Seattle, Washington:

I remember that I was running downstairs because I knew that the war had started. Outside, there was the sound of a siren, and

I could see men and women running through the streets. The stairs were covered in smashed-up crackers, which didn't make it very easy to run down. I clung on to a picture on the wall, but it broke to pieces in my hands, and I fell end over end down the stairs until I landed on the sidewalk.

There was a woman running towards me with six or seven howling dogs on a leash. She was nude. She looked very angry and said: 'Where have you been? We're fighting already. This way!' I ran after her down the street, and we arrived in a kind of plaza. It was waist-deep in prickly plants, and there were thirty or maybe forty naked women standing amongst the plants, shooting rifles at a big marble building on one side of the plaza. They were breaking all the windows. There didn't seem to be anybody in the building itself to return the shooting.

I had to run through the prickly plants. I was naked, too, and it was very painful. I crouched down in case someone shot me. I said to one of the girls: 'Where are my clothes?' and she said: 'Are you a woman or aren't you? Who invented clothes, and what for?' I didn't know whether I knew the answer to that. But then another siren blew, and we all had to run into this huge marble building, and hundreds of naked girls were swarming up the stairs, waving flags and shrieking at the tops of their voices.

We forced our way into a huge conference room or banqueting hall, and the whole place was stacked high with the corpses of naked men. I didn't know what to do. I said to one of the girls who was with me: 'Is this the right way to do it?'

Then the dream seemed to change. There was still some kind of war going on. But it was more like the First War. I was naked, but I had a flowery hat on, and thigh-length silk stockings with flowery garters. I was standing in a huge railroad station, and I think it was Grand Central in New York, but I'm not altogether sure. There were sounds like elephants trumpeting, and I knew that those must be the trains. I was looking for someone. A man. I saw someone that I thought must be him. He was wearing an army uniform and he was smoking a cigar. I went over but it wasn't him at all. I had to climb on to one of the trains to see if I could find him. I looked frantically in every compartment. I knew the train was going to leave at any moment, and I would have to get off.

At last I found him, at the end of one of the corridors, leaning out of the window. I don't know who the man was, because I didn't see his face very clearly. His cap made such a dark shadow over his eyes. I clung to him and kissed him. He opened up his army coat, and he fucked me, then and there, standing up in the train corridor. I didn't even have an orgasm, but he managed to shoot his stuff inside me. The train was moving, and I wanted to get off. He said I had to stay. It was too late. He said: 'You're fighting with me now, but it won't always be this way. One day you'll fight against me, and I'm worried that you're going to win.'

The woman who dreamed this dream was not committed to women's liberation in the sense that she felt she belonged to an army of militant ladies. She was aware of the existence of the Women's Lib movement, and (as her dream showed) she was sympathetic to its causes. But there was a sense of being an *outsider* in this dream, a sense of being reluctant to attack men as a means of winning freedom.

The 'war' that opened her dream was the war between men and women. So many magazines and newspapers have used the phrase 'The Battle of the Sexes' that it isn't surprising that the conflict emerged in her dream as a full-scale blitzkrieg. Sirens were blowing (there may have been police sirens in the street outside while she slept), and there was a sense of danger and urgency. She ran downstairs. The stairs were blocked with smashed crackers, and she was able to interpret this image for herself.

'My Uncle Ted was the messiest saltine eater I ever came across. I have an image in my mind of seeing him when I was a kid, and there he was, shedding his crumbs all over his vest. He was also very chauvinistic, and I guess that the smashed crackers in the dream were a little reminder of him.'

As she ran outside, she met a fierce nude woman with howling dogs. There are countless pictures of this woman in classical mythology, and this was one time when I felt the archetypal dream image was the right one. This was

Diana, the huntress, the powerful independent figure of militant feminine revenge. Sure enough, her army of feminist soldiers are besieging a building (the Male Establishment) and breaking its windows.

The meaning of the prickly plants in the square never became entirely clear. They may have represented the difficulties she felt she had to go through to win her womanly independence. 'Prickly' has distinct connotations of 'pricks' and 'penises'. They may have represented nothing at all but a sense of physical discomfort. She made a note of the plants, and made up her mind to check them again if she ever had more dreams about them.

There was a dream conversation about the necessity of clothes. She wasn't consciously aware that she had ever felt that clothes were invented by men to make women into sexually attractive objects. But she did have some sympathy with women who thought the ever-changing dictates of fashion were an expensive and occasionally demeaning imposition on women's anxiety.

Finally, the building was taken. The men were defeated. But she was shocked to find them all dead. She didn't believe that the price of female freedom should be male distress. 'After all,' she said. 'I'm not the Valerie Solanas of Seattle.'

It was this thought, in my opinion, that led her to go into the second stage of the dream, the First War stage. She was no longer militant in this part of the dream, nor involved in militant behavior. She was still naked, but the nakedness was not a symbol of feminine independence anymore. It was cute, flowery, erotic nakedness – 'the kind men like.' Her position in relation to men had altered. The man (and I don't think he was any special man, but just a typical man) was the dominant force. He was off to the war, off to do all the aggressive and active and masculine things that men do. She was staying behind – inferior and feminine and only there for a last quick fuck. The dream was explaining why she felt the way she did about feminine liberation. It was because she felt used by men, and under-appreciated. She was having trouble with her work at the swimpool because her boss considered that women were incompetent by definition, and she was also having trouble with her boyfriend, who treated her with great offhandedness.

But there was a glimmer of hope in the dream. The soldier said: 'One day you'll fight against me ... and you're going to win.' Since her own dreaming mind created these words, it's possible that she felt, deep down, that she did have a chance of getting her own way. That was one reason why she shouldn't ignore the dream. It was telling her a lot about herself and what her future could be like if she took advantage of her character and her potential.

Trains and railroad stations appear in a great many sexual dreams, both male and female. This may partly be due to the romantic image that most people have of railroads (except those people who have recently suffered the ministrations of AmTrak), and partly due to their phallic appearance. But many dreams involve travel and a sense of going someplace. This is the way in which dreams illustrate the passing of time, and the development of human affairs.

You will see from the way in which we have interpreted these ten dreams that your own memories, associations, and inspirations are essential to good analysis. You will see, too, that dream interpretation is a long and sometimes complicated business. The best that I have been able to do here is discuss some of the more obvious themes of the ten dreams, and it would take pages of print to describe all the thinking and suggestions that should usually go into your own interpretations.

Erotic dreams have to be interpreted on several different

levels. Some of the meanings of your dreams will come to you in a flash, and you will know exactly what you've been dreaming about straightaway. But other meanings – even within the same dream that you've begun to solve so quickly – will take hours and even days of applied thought. Once you've come to a complicated impasse, don't try to hurry your dream interpretation along. The more time you spend on it, the clearer your final interpretation is likely to be. There is no harm in the 'instant' analysis, provided you understand that it will need to be changed and reshaped as you probe further into the details of your dream. Don't ever let yourself accept a dream interpretation that you know is not really 'right'. Even if you can't solve the meaning of one dream, it's likely that you will dream about the same situation again in a different way, and next time you may be able to interpret it more easily.

Earlier on, I mentioned recent dream research which has shown that women's dreams are affected by their menstrual cycle. This notably affects your erotic dreams. As you've probably realized for yourself, your sexual drive waxes and wanes throughout your menstrual month, and your physical and mental condition is bound to alter what you dream about. Different women are affected in different ways. When you're keeping an erotic dream diary, make sure that you note down the passing of your menstrual cycle alongside the dreams, so that you can see when you have had each dream in relation to your period. After a few months, you will begin to notice a pattern in the contents of your sexual dreams – a pattern that is detectably related to your physical rhythms.

'Halfway through my period,' a 34-year-old Texas woman told me, 'I have dream after dream of sex. I feel like making love all day long, and I keep having these amazing dreams. Every period, it's the same.'

There may be other cycles that affect your erotic dreams,

too, but you will probably only discover these if you keep your diary for a very long time. Some women are affected by the seasons, others by pregnancy. One woman from Illinois even claimed she used to have erotic dreams at regular six-week intervals, because years ago her husband used to have six-week leaves from his job on a large construction site in Alaska!

So little is known about dreams – so little is known about you – that your erotic dream interpretations will be breaking completely new ground. As we've seen, only you can supply a definitive analysis. But the erotic dream lexicon that follows will act as a guide, and give you some ideas that may lead you out of the woods when you get lost. It's not a dream dictionary in the sense that you simply look something up – say 'fat men' or 'horses' penises' or 'cucumbers' – and immediately find out what you've really been dreaming about. No dictionary can tell you that, and any dictionary that claims it can is a fraud.

This lexicon was especially prepared for the sexual dreams of women – one of the very few that ever has been. Interpret your dream by yourself as best you can, and then turn to the lexicon to give yourself inspiration for further analysis. Provided you're honest with yourself, and you use the lexicon as a list of suggestions rather than a definitive dictionary, you should be able to discover new and fascinating paths through the dark and complex forest of your sexual personality.

BOOK TWO
A Lexicon of Women's Erotic Dreams

A

Abduction

Being abducted is a favorite female fantasy dream and is often associated with romantic images and excitement. These dreams are rarely realistic in themselves, but they usually happen for a very realistic reason. They show that you're dissatisfied with your present sexual life, and you're looking for a way out – or at least an improvement. You don't, however, have the necessary strength to make the decision yourself. You're looking for Rudolph Valentino to come galloping past the A&P and sweep you off on his white charger.

I was sitting in the park with my baby daughter when a band of naked, savage-looking men, all armed with swords and decorated with bracelets and rings, seized hold of me and started to drag me away. One of them picked Miranda up and took her along, too, so I wasn't too worried. They carried me over their heads into a kind of white palace. They lowered me down to the floor, and they literally tore the clothes off my back. Then they took me towards a throne, where a young prince was sitting. I had to kneel on the marble floor, and stretch right back until my head was touching the tiles behind me. Then the prince came down from his throne, handed his clothes to his servants, and made love to me. He was brown and young, and he smelled of Eastern perfumes. He made love like an angel. I can remember thinking how wonderful this all was, and how my life was going to start all over again. He waited until I had had seven or eight orgasms, and then he thrust into me quicker and quicker, and his come felt red-hot inside me, like drops of molten metal. I was just about to say something to him when I woke up.

When you have a dream like this, take a good look at yourself and your mate. Are you having enough sex? Is your partner dominant enough, decisive enough? Could you coax him into mending his ways? Or are you going to start looking for someone new?

Adultery

If you have erotic dreams of adultery, they don't necessarily mean that you have real adultery on your mind. But adultery dreams are usually 'warning' dreams — they're telling you that you're dissatisfied with your current sex relationships, and that, consciously or unconsciously, you're looking around for something or someone new. Often, the dream itself will give you a clue about what kind of problem you're suffering from, as in this dream from a 28-year-old housewife:

I dreamed I was at home, lying on the bed. I had my nightie on, but I pulled it up right to my waist. The door opened and my next-door neighbor walked in. He was carrying his cock in his hand, and he was smiling. He screwed his cock into place, just like the handle of a pair of garden shears, and he came over to the bed and stared at me, playing with his cock all the time. He said I had a beautiful cunt, and he wanted to fuck me. I went all silly and saucy and said: 'Go ahead.' I pulled open the lips of my cunt, and he bent down and took a look. He nodded, and said: 'Oh yes. You're only getting it once a week, aren't you?' I blushed. I didn't know how he could know that. He climbed on top of me and fucked me in a very strange and unsatisfying way, then he got up and left.

It was obvious from this dream that the girl had no real desire to have sex with her neighbor. But she was feeling frustrated since she only had intercourse once a week, and her dream, was diagnosing the trouble for her. Since she knew that her husband would never admit he wasn't virile enough to keep her happy, the diagnosis had to come from another man. In her dream, she felt obliged to have sex with him, but she didn't enjoy it at all. If you have dreams like this, then take a good look at your sexual relationship and ask yourself if it's as good as it could be. One of the great things about dreams is that they do give you plenty of warning of impending problems.

Airplane

Airplanes are phallic but they are also womb-like, because they are hollow and they contain people. Depending on whether you dream about the inside or the outside of the airplane, your dream may indicate that you are thinking about the progress of your sexual relationship with a man or with a woman. All vessels, like boats and cars and buses, have bisexual characteristics. That doesn't mean that you are necessarily bisexual if you dream about them, but it does mean that your dream is considering the influence of both a man and a woman on your sexual life. Airplanes usually represent a keen sense of progress at speed. Perhaps you're worried about the short duration of your current sexual relationship. Perhaps you're looking for escape. For most people, erotic dreams which include airplanes are dreams which underline the dangerous and precarious nature of their present sexual situation. For a fuller interpretation of airplanes, see *1,001 Erotic Dreams Interpreted*.

Animals

If you have sexual dreams in which animals appear, you may be dreaming about your own erotic desires or the desires of someone you are close to. When you see your sexual lusts as animals, it's because you are fundamentally ashamed of them, and if you dream that you are fighting the animals, then you may be going through an internal conflict with your passions. Here is an interesting animal dream that makes the point clear:

I was sitting on a leopard-skin settee in a room full of mirrors. A friend of my father's was sitting opposite me. He was wearing a black suit, and he was stroking a vicious-looking lion creature, about the size of a large tomcat. When I looked closely, I felt excited by the way the tomcat was looking at me, but I also realized that my father's friend's suit was covered in hairs that the animal had shed.

The 'lion creature' represented this girl's own sexual desire for her father's friend, a sexual desire which she had previously suppressed. It may also have represented the desire which he had shown for her, but which she hadn't wanted to recognize. The way the animal shed its hairs could have meant that she was worried her desire would be seen and discovered. Dreams of shedding hair and teeth also represent a sense of loss and sexual frigidity. If you dream you are having sex with animals, your dream interpretation will depend on the animal (consult this lexicon for the meaning of particular beasts) and the way you feel about making love to it. The animal may represent a particular person you know, seen in terms of their animal lusts instead of their usual human form, or it may represent your own lusts. Most dreams in which women have sex with animals have some masochistic content – a desire to be humiliated and to derive some erotic excitement out of sexual self-abasement.

I dreamed I was nude, tied up in a stable. I was filthy and covered in dung and mud. There was a huge black stallion in the stable with me, and my father and my brother led him up to me. They raised my legs in the air, and while my brother kept my thighs apart, my father coaxed the stallion's enormous penis into me. I adored it. I screamed out for more. I wanted the horse's penis in further. I wanted it in right up to its big greasy balls. I didn't care how disgusting I was, or what I did.

This was the erotic dream of a girl who had just begun her first affair at the age of 18. She came from a tightly knit, religious farming family, and her dream was a visualization of how she felt about herself sexually. She was half aroused and excited by her discovery of sexual feelings, and half guilty because her background had led her to believe that sex was dirty and animalistic. She had also seen the stallions around her father's spread, and had secretly wondered about their sexual organs before. The dream does not mean that the girl is ever likely to make love to a horse for real, or that there is anything psychologically wrong with her. If you dream of training animals, you are possibly trying to get your sexual feelings under control. If you dream of kissing and cuddling animals, you are at peace with your sexuality, and you are likely to be a very affectionate and sexy girl. If you dream of strange animals you have never seen before, you may be uncertain about the true character of your sexual personality. If you dream of riding animals, you are a strong-willed and sensual woman who has her sexuality under strict control. As a general rule, animals represent people who exhibit similar personal behavior (dogs — faithful and diffident; mice — timid and shy). Animals may talk in your dreams, which is a sure sign that they are symbolizing someone you know.

Appetites

When you are hungry or thirsty in your sexual dreams, this may well mean that you are lusting for sexual satisfaction. Freud believed that our appetites often appear in less embarrassing guises in our dreams, and many dreams in which women crave food or water in sexually suggestive circumstances seem to back him up. Eating and drinking are very closely associated with sex (remember the orgiastic eating scene in the movie *Tom Jones*, in which Tom seduces his *amour* with his less-than-innocent ingestion of a chicken leg). This is particularly true since oral sexual techniques have received wider publicity and acceptability. Here's a short dream which clarifies the way in which appetites can be interchangeable:

I am sitting watching television with my boyfriend. I begin to feel terribly hungry. I kiss him, and I whisper in his ear that I'm hungry. He nods. He walked out of the room and comes back with a strange shiny-looking hamburger. I open my mouth wide and force the hamburger straight in. I feel as if I'm going to choke. I can't breathe. But then I have an extraordinary sexual climax, and the hamburger slides down.

The girl was able to interpret this dream fairly easily herself. She had recently been reading Linda Lovelace's autobiography, and the 'hamburger' scene was her own euphemistic attempt to deep-throat her boyfriend. Check, when you've been having dreams of thirst or hunger, that you simply weren't hungry or thirsty when you went to bed. Real sensations can often permeate through to your dreams.

Ascending

If you dream of going upwards in an elevator, or you dream of climbing stairs, you may be dreaming of sexual intercourse, or of trying to improve your sexual technique. Freud believed that staircases could represent the vaginal passage, although you will have to decide for yourself whether they mean the same to you. If you dream of climbing stairs with a man you find attractive, you may be considering sexual relations with him since 'let's go upstairs' is a common euphemism for 'let's go to bed and have sex.' If you never reach the top of the stairs, you may be recognizing the fact that you'll never make it with this particular man, or that considerable difficulties stand in your way. A dream of trying to ascend an endless staircase on your own may represent your repeated attempts to reach orgasm without success. Look closely at other details within the dream to see if they give you clues about the reasons for your failure.

B

Bag

Erotic dreams which include bags or purses or pocket-books are often saying something about your vagina. One woman actually had a dream in which she caught her husband having sex with her alligator handbag. Bags with things in them (money, food, etc) may represent what you hope to get out of your sexual relationships. You may feel that you are prostituting yourself at the present time, and that you are giving sex in return for favors. The bag is more likely to represent a vagina if it has vaginal characteristics (tight, stretchy, soft).

Balls

When your erotic dreams are about balls, you may be dreaming about your lover or your husband and his sexual virility. Dreams are always having little jokes and making little puns, and to turn a man's testicles into billiard balls or ball bearings or eggs is a typical dream device. If you dream about balls in association with pregnancy dreams, then you are almost certainly dreaming about your mate's potency. If you dream about handling delicate balls with great care, you may be worried about your sexual technique and the delicacy of your partner's sexual organs.

I had a dream, and in this dream I took my husband's penis right down my throat. He took it out again, but I found I had two big round hard candies left in my mouth, one tucked into each cheek. I kept trying to look between my husband's legs, to see if I'd sucked them out by mistake, but he wouldn't sit in the right way, to allow me to see. When I sucked the candies, they had the exact salty-bitter taste of my husband's sperm, and I knew that I'd swallowed his balls by accident. I was quite interested, though, about what I'd found out. I never knew a man's balls were made of solid sperm, like candy.

That was the dream of a 22-year-old newlywed who had tried to be as sexually adventurous as possible after reading a fairly advanced sex technique book. Her adventurousness was not matched by her sexual knowledge, and she was sometimes afraid she was doing the wrong thing. But that wasn't disastrous. Her dream was only reminding her that she didn't quite know everything there was to know about sex just yet. She would soon find out. Balls can also represent breasts or pregnant stomachs.

Bananas

To dream about eating bananas is often a thinly veiled dream of fellatio (sucking your lover's penis). But a banana can't talk or answer back, so your dream may be telling you that you prefer your sex without any personalities or problems attached.

Bells

Deep, tolling bells can be a warning of sexual dangers. A New York woman dreamed she was having sex with her best friend's husband. She enjoyed it, but she was worried by the persistent clanging of a bell in the distance. Bells of this kind, associated as they are with alarms and churches, can be a nagging reminder that what you're doing is morally dubious, and may not be in your own best interests. Tinkling bells and merry bells are much more likely to represent sexual delight and happiness. They may also express an unconscious desire to marry. Generally, though, bells represent an interruption of your sexual indulgence by your conscience.

Birds

Birds often appear in dreams, and the ancient dream interpreters set great store by them. Crows looked like priests and, therefore, represented death; owls were the departed souls of the dead; wild geese were the pagan divinities who accompanied witches; phoenixes represented resurrection; and cocks represented lust. If you dream about seeing flying birds in the distance, you may be dreaming about your sexual aspirations and wishes for ecstasy. You may also be dreaming about sending messages to someone you love. If you dream about caged birds, you are feeling frustrated in your sex life, and you are looking for a way to express the sexual personality you know you have. If you dream about peacocks, and other birds with magnificent plumage, you may be dreaming about sexual display and deliberate showing-off – either by yourself or by someone you know. Hens and chickens represent utilitarian, earthbound people and ideas. If you have dreams of chickens, you may either wish to see yourself in a permanent domestic role, or, more likely, you are worried that you are no longer considered by your husband or lover to be a sexy and romantic person. Birds passing overhead can represent the passage of time in dreams, and birds disappearing can represent a vanishing relationship.

In my dream, I had to play a game with two men. We balanced on big red balls, like circus people, all over a smooth grassy field. I can't remember what the point of the game was, but in the dream I understood it. I think I won. When this had happened, the game was over. One man stood in front of me, and the other stood behind me. The man behind me held on to the cheeks of my bottom and skewered his hard cock right up my ass. I could feel his pubic hair in the cleft of my bottom, like electric fuse wire. The other man, in front of me, he held on to my shoulders and pushed his cock into my pussy. The two of them held hands, and dropped us all over on to our sides on the grass. Then we rolled faster and faster down a slope, and the feeling was more than just orgasmic. I mean, it was so sexy that I was screaming and shrieking out loud. I was coming and I was shitting myself at the same time. When it was over, the men had turned into geese. I couldn't understand it. They spoke just like men, but they had turned into geese. They flapped their wings, and then they flew off. I watched them disappear into the distance. I felt an awful sense of loneliness.

This was the sexual dream of a 26-year-old Seattle girl who was breaking off a long-standing affair with her boyfriend. Both men were different aspects of her boyfriend's personality, and her dream had divided him into two. But the net result was the same. He turned into birds and left her. The goose, as ancient dream diviners have told us, is one of the most self-willed and intractable of characters and can fly away over sea, land, or anyplace at all.

Bites

Sexual dreams which involve biting — no matter how vicious and aggressive that biting may be — are usually dreams of extreme erotic affection. There may be some cruelty involved in your sexual relationship, but it's obviously a relationship of devouring passion and lust. Either that, or you're wishing that it were. If you dream that you bite off your husband's or lover's penis, you're still showing your love and not your desire to emasculate him. Dreams of biting off penises usually haunt young girls who have tried fellatio for the first time and are worried that they're going to hurt their boyfriends accidentally. If you dream that you bite off your lover's penis and *eat* it, however, you may have unconscious desires to acquire some of his qualities and characteristics. You may still admire and love him, but you may feel that you want some of the masculine confidence and strength that he's got.

Blood

In sexual dreams, blood can represent menstrual blood, or it can represent male sperm. You will probably be able to tell which from the context in which it appears. To dream of vampires or bloodsucking is highly sexual, and represents oral intercourse (hence, the way in which women swoon with ecstasy when Dracula makes a meal of their offside necks). Dreaming of open wounds which refuse to stop bleeding is usually indicative of anxiety about menstruation. If you dream of wounds which *refuse* to bleed, you may be concerned that you're pregnant. Don't push it to the back of your mind – admit how worried you really are. Should you dream of drinking a man's blood, you are toying with the thought of intimate sexual acts with him, specifically fellatio. If you dream of drinking a woman's blood, you may be trying to destroy her, and at the same time acquire for yourself her sexual charms and power.

Body

Some dream diviners claim that the various parts of your body can represent different situations, attitudes, and objects. Hands and limbs can represent the penis. The right side of your body can represent your upright, moral qualities, and the left side of your body can represent your lusts and your failings. I have yet to see any evidence of these interpretations, but they might work for you. Several dreams which feature earholes and nostrils and even eye-sockets have obvious sexual implications; the women who dreamed them seem to be embarrassed about their sexual organs, and so they dreamed about another part of them-selves. As one Cleveland woman said: 'I dreamed my lover came to me with his penis sticking out. I took out my left eye and he pushed his penis into the hole. It was sheer ecstasy. He was making love to me right into my mind. I felt the relationship was so much more constructive because it was *mental* as well as physical. I don't like to feel like an *animal*.' Don't be alarmed by the vision of being fucked in the eye. As we've seen before, dreams are not as sadistic as they sometimes appear to be. Tom Chetwynd, in his *Dictionary for Dreamers*, mentions that if you dream of having something stuck in your eye, it may mean that you are dreaming of coitus.

Book

If books appear in your sexual dreams, you may be thinking back over past affairs. Books, according to ancient diviners, indicate memories and regrets.

Breasts

Like penises and vaginas, breasts appear in erotic dreams in all sorts of extraordinary ways. Sometimes they're hard, like oranges or apples, and sometimes they're as soft and malleable as modeling clay. In erotic dreams, your dream breasts are very often bigger than your own breasts actually are, and this is an indication of the importance that our society, artistically and culturally, has placed on the enormous breast. Sexiness = big boobs. While this has no foundation in any kind of fact at all, many women still profess that they feel sexier when they have large breasts (especially small-breasted women during pregnancy). If you persistently dream about your breasts, you may be pondering over some minor anxiety you have about them. Are they too big, too small? Do you think they're a funny shape? But it depends on how you dream about them. If you're displaying them openly to other people, you may be trying to show the world that you're sexier than they seem to think you are. If you're fondling and squeezing your own breasts, you are turning your attention to your own sexual stimulation, and you may be feeling that your lover doesn't pay your breasts enough attention when you make love. If your breasts grow to gigantic proportions, you are possibly displaying your femininity to the point of being ludicrous about it, and your dream may be warning you that you are acting too provocative for your own good. Dreams of baring your breasts in public may also be associated with your involvement in women's liberation (if you have any), and your feelings that women's most obvious physical difference is there to be displayed and appreciated. A Nevada go-go dancer came out with this dream when she was undergoing silicone pad enlargement of her bust:

I had the most giant boobs in the whole universe, right? They were giant. If I stretched both my arms out in front of me, I could just about touch my nipples. Because they weren't soft, these boobs. They were hard and they stuck up way in front of me. I knew I was the sexiest girl in the whole universe. I was strutting my stuff along the sidewalk with a real tight dress on, and high heels, and these giant boobs.

She said that she would like to have had boobs like that for real – which shows how deeply the idea of 'sexiness = big boobs' has become implanted in our sexual culture. If you dream of a baby sucking at your breasts, and you're deriving sexual pleasure from it, you may be dreaming of the complete sexual satisfaction of having a child, or you may be dreaming that you are giving sexual pleasure to your lover or husband. If a man is less experienced and less powerful than you in personality, then it's not uncommon for him to seem physically smaller in your dreams.

Bull

The bull is a symbol of rampant masculinity from times of antiquity, and it still has those associations today. If you have an erotic dream in which a bull appears, there may be a man in your life who is forceful and sexual, but whose sheer masculine aggressiveness tends to intimidate you. Remember that the bull is evil tempered and domineering as well as sexually powerful, and that people who stray into a bull's field often have to run for their lives. If you dream of being gored by a bull, or having a bull's horn penetrating your vagina, you are probably dreaming that this dominant masculine character is having his way with you. Think back over how you felt when it happened. Frightened? Pleased? Excited? Anxious? Those feelings will tell you what you really think of the man in question, and you can then act accordingly.

C

Cat

Cats, when they appear in your erotic dreams, almost invariably have associations with the powerful and mystical side of womanhood. They are worshipped as gods in ancient Egypt, and they still represent sensuality, feline independence, and impenetrable feminine secrecy. Your interpretation will depend on the cat itself, and how you feel about cats. Remember that it could be a dream pun for your 'pussy', particularly if it is explicitly involved in any sexual scenes.

Cinema

If you have a dream in which you are sitting in a cinema watching a sex film, take heed of what is happening on the screen. Your mind is sitting you down for the specific purpose of telling you something about your sex life. It may also be hinting that you are too detached about your erotic relationships, and that you are something of a watcher rather than a participant. A 24-year-old Chicago girl dreamed that:

I was sitting in the movies watching the dirtiest movie you ever saw in your whole life. I can't remember much of it. There was a scene where a girl took six stiff dicks into her mouth at once, and then blew out about a gallon of white sperm. There was another scene where a girl had been raped up the ass, and they showed a real close-up. Stuff like that, I didn't even realize I knew anything about. But during the whole movie a guy was sitting next to me, and he had his hand right up my dress, and he was diddling my clitoris with his finger. It was definitely the rudest dream I can ever recall.

This dream was simply showing the girl that she was not doing enough in her sexual relationship to satisfy her lover. She suspected it during her waking hours but had never been able to admit it to herself so frankly. The man who sat next to her in her dream, masturbating her, was so anonymous that he may have been a part of her own sexual character — the aloof, detached part that would rather seek her own pleasures and avoid involvement with other people. If you dream you are watching a comedy while you are having sex — whether it's movies or TV — you may feel that your sex life is rather ludicrous and gauche.

Cliff

If you have a sexual dream in which you are making love close to the edge of a cliff or precipice, you may be anxious that your present relationship is about to come to an abrupt and nasty conclusion. Women who have difficulty in reaching orgasm have told me that they sometimes have dreams of cliffs — walking to the brink, almost as if they were hypnotically drawn by the prospect of plunging over, only to find that they can't.

Climax

Sexual climaxes are a totally subjective experience, and everybody perceives them in a different way. In sexual dreams, however, climaxes don't just seem to be individual and varied. They are bizarre and colorful and take many eccentric forms and shapes. Sometimes they take the form of achievement in a favorite *nonsexual* pastime, like this dream from a 31-year-old Washington, DC, woman:

It was evening and we were playing tennis on the lawns. The sun was low in the sky. I was playing with my husband, and we were both playing beautifully. I found that I could leap up to incredible heights to reach the ball, and that my raquet was like a living thing in my hand. At first, we started playing slow and languorous, but after a while we began to play really fast and furious, running and leaping from one side of the court to the other. I played like a dream the whole time, and I couldn't help thinking how well my husband and I were moving together, what beautiful rhythms we had. Towards the end of the game we were playing so fast that people could hardly see us. I leaped up into the sky to backhand the ball, seven or eight feet into the evening air, and I suddenly understood that I was having an orgasm. I almost exploded in mid-air, it was like my whole being was coming apart. And then I sank slowly back to the lawn, the same way that a feather sinks, and I never felt so happy and contented in my whole life.

This dream has some interesting parallels with some of the dreams in the late Jack Kerouac's *Book of Dreams*, in which he imagined he was playing baseball with amazing agility and made tremendous moon-like leaps into the air. If you dream about having orgasms, it may well be an indication that you are sexually fulfilled, but climax dreams are often more complex than that. Try and define what the climax was like. Was there anything unusual about it? Or was there some strange object or person present when you were having your climax that throws some relevant light on it? One Vermont woman dreamed that, whenever she had an orgasm, an awful green glazed pot was in the room, standing on an ugly little table. She was eventually able to interpret the presence of the pot, which had once belonged to her mother, as a sign of her parents' disapproval at her living with her boyfriend and the sexual guilt she felt because of their disapproval. In other words, every moment of sexual satisfaction was accompanied by an ugly presence, an awkward doubt. If you dream that your climaxes are like fiery explosions, then you may unconsciously believe that your present sexual relationship is too passionate and volatile to last for very long. If you dream that your climaxes are like liquid, or make you feel like liquid, then you may be showing how acquiescent and passive you are during sex. There is a suggestion, too, that you might have strong maternal feelings about the sexual act: The sea and other liquids are very feminine, motherly images, and it was the biological melting-pot of the ocean which gave birth to human life. Hundreds of ancient dream interpretations mention the sea as a birthplace, as a fecund but domineering mother. If you dream that your climaxes make you very light and buoyant, you may be the kind of woman who looks to sex for escape from reality. It might be better to face your problems squarely, and not seek momentary oblivion in sex and other escapist entertainments. If your climax makes you feel heavy and dense, you are displaying the deep intensity of your sexual passions, but you are also showing how seriously you take the responsibility of a sexual liaison. Some women dream their orgasms in dominant colors: red, green, blue, etc. If you do, consult the entry on colors in this lexicon and see whether it makes your climax dream easier to understand.

Clitoris

Although the clitoris exactly corresponds to the male penis, women dream about it in a very different way. The trouble is that, despite its sexual importance, it's tucked away out of sight, and you have to use mirrors and open your legs if you want to take a good look at it. Men will often dream about the penis as a stick or a rod, or just as a penis, but women dream about the clitoris in all kinds of weird guises – simply because they have no clear idea of what it looks like. Here's a typical example, from a 25-year-old Dallas, Texas, woman:

I dreamed I went to the doctor. There was something wrong with my clitoris, and he was going to have to examine it. He made me lie down on his couch, and then he took down my panties and opened my thighs and stared at me. I colored up, I was so embarrassed. But at the same time, it was quite erotic to have another man look at me so close. After awhile, he told me that he'd found out what the trouble was. He produced this thing from out of my vagina that looked exactly like a fat pink chili. He rubbed it between his finger and his thumb, and it gave me a beautiful sexy feeling. Then he put it into his mouth and sucked it, and I was feeling faint all over, I was so turned-on. Then he swallowed it. I said: 'What have you done? You've swallowed my clitoris.' He said: 'That's okay. Here's a script for another one.' But I wasn't sure if he was maybe lying or not.

If you dream you have an enormous, penis-like clitoris, you may have latent desires to take a more leading and aggressive role in your sexual relationships. If you cannot locate your clitoris in your dream, you may be unsure of your sexual personality and your sexual confidence, and you are fumbling for the right way to find erotic fulfillment.

Colors

Everybody dreams in full color, with a few notable exceptions. Colors are often excellent clues to the meaning of your erotic dreams, because they represent your feelings and your passions in strong and visual terms. Here's a dream from a 21-year-old New Orleans girl which shows how important color can be:

I dreamed I was running naked through a meadow. The grass was vivid green, and I felt happy and very carefree. There was some black-and-white cows in the distance, and they were eating the grass, grazing. I felt worried about them for some reason. I stopped running and started to walk, staring at the cows. While I was walking, my boyfriend jumped out from behind a hedge.

He had a long stick, like a cop's nightstick, and he started to run after me waving this stick. I knew I had to run past the black-and-white cows and I was afraid. I didn't know whether I ought to risk being butted by the cows, or let my boyfriend catch up with me. In the end, I pretended to trip. My boyfriend caught me, and held me upside down by my heels. I was kicking and struggling. I knew he could see right into my vagina, and I didn't want him to. He bent me over double, and then he had his penis out, and he practically raped me. I thought he was going to split me, his penis seemed so big. But then I had an orgasm, and he let me go. He gave me a dirty sheet to cover myself with, and we went home.

Interpreting the colors in this dream alone, we can discover that the girl feels happy, innocent, carefree, and full of vitality (green); but she feels internal conflict about sex (black-and-white); she has intercourse with her boyfriend, and afterwards she feels soiled (dirty white). Colors can represent many things, from the obvious *yellow = cowardice* and *red = anger* to quite complicated meanings that are based on the holy colors of ancient religions. As a general rule, red is associated with strong feelings, with blood and fire and passion; white is associated with sexual purity and innocence (although white fluids represent semen); purple is associated with virility and sexual strength; lilac with failing sexual vigor and even death; yellow with erotic exhibitionism (and yellow liquids with urine); brown with feelings of lust and earthy passions, also with excrement; black with maternal feelings; blue with devotion, faithfulness, and singlemindedness; gold with masculinity; silver with femininity; green with growth and friendship. Of course, these definitions of the meanings of colors in sexual dreams are not always relevant to what you've dreamed about. Red or black may have particular associations for you which you alone can know about. But they are based on both modern psychological research and on ancient dream books, and they are a fair summing-up of whatever knowledge there is about the significance of colors in dreams. I believe that colors are so important, in fact, that it is worthwhile for you to go through a whole dream in nothing but its basic colors to see what they mean to you. From my own experience with magazine sales, I found that magazines with blue covers always sold more than magazines with yellow covers. Any market research expert will tell you that we respond very impulsively and emotionally to colors, and this, in my view, makes it inevitable that our sexual dreams should be colored according to our erotic feelings. Try and work out your own color code, and include it in your erotic dream diary.

Crown

Dreaming of wearing a crown on your head when you are having sex is an indication that you are pleased with your sexual success and your sexual attractiveness, and you feel you have achieved something worthwhile in your intimate relationships. If your lover is wearing a crown, you could be seeking a father-figure in your sex life or someone who will take charge of your sex life for you — initiating sex acts and telling you what to do.

Cunnilingus

Men who have dreams about cunnilingus are usually stable, well-oriented lovers who have no fears about the female sexual organs and how to stimulate them. But women who have repeated dreams about men licking their vaginas are looking for something different. They may be looking for subservient behavior from the men in their lives or for recognition that they are proud, haughty, and attractive ladies. Cunnilingus dreams, while they have elements of domination and submission, are not sadistic. One Massachusetts girl even dreamed that when her lover licked her vulva, it flowed with wine, and he was able to have an alcoholic evening without even leaving the bedroom. It is possible to dream that another girl is giving you cunnilingus, or that you are giving cunnilingus to another girl, without having secret lesbian tendencies. Many subtle shades of relationship are represented in dreams by blatant and obvious activities, particularly when it comes to sex, and you are probably dreaming that you are showing your admiration for her, or that she is showing her admiration for you. That is, unless there is further evidence in your sexual dreams that you have lesbian undercurrents beneath the surface of your erotic personality.

D

Death

Erotic dreams in which death occurs are very seldom concerned with real death. If you dream about your lover dying, then (depending on your reaction to it) you are probably expressing your anxiety that your relationship is growing cold and fading away and also expressing your aggressive feelings toward your lover because he doesn't show you the same affection that he used to. In ancient times, dreams of death were considered to be good omens, and a sign that the dreamer was going to get whatever he wanted out of life. Sometimes, dreams of death are purely circumstantial: Tom Chetwynd mentions a woman who dreamed that a relative had died, just so that she could go to the funeral and have another glimpse of the man she loved. Death dreams can warn you of your frigid feelings for the man in your life or that you are seeking too much sympathy from your lover (many suicides, after all, are only trying to attract attention to themselves). This dream of death from a 30-year-old Milwaukee woman is very curious:

I dreamed my lover had died. My husband never knew about my lover, and so I had to pretend that I was going out to the supermarket when I went down to look at my lover lying in the funeral parlor. He was lying in a coffin with his shirt and tuxedo jacket on. His face was very white. His eyes were shut. I looked closer, and saw that he wasn't wearing any pants. His penis was sticking up rigid. I took hold of it, and found that I could unscrew it, quite easy, like a light bulb. There was a piece of paper inside it with a message. The message was in a strange language I couldn't read, but I knew that it meant he wasn't dead, and if I hurried down to the (then) Sheraton Schroeder, he would meet me in the bar, and we'd fly off to San Francisco together.

For this woman, her lover's apparent death was a way of escaping from the real world, where she had to live with her husband, and making the perfect getaway. I like the image of the screw-off penis with the message inside. It came from a TV movie she had recently seen, in which a pirate had secreted a treasure-map inside his wooden leg.

Depths

If you have sexual dreams in which you are deep in the earth or the sea, then you may be having powerful dreams about your sexual character and your womanliness. Time and time again, ancient and modern dream interpretations show that deep, formless, all-embracing situations represent womanhood. Depending on whether you are secure in the depths or afraid of their overwhelming weight, your dream will tell you whether you're comfortable with your sexual identity or anxious about it. If you dream you have lost your way in deep caves, or if you dream that you're drowning, you may be searching for some way of understanding your femininity and relating it to the outside world – particularly to the man you love.

Desert

If your sexual dream takes place in a desert, then you may be feeling isolated from other people by your sexual actions and your sexual desires. Deserts sometimes represent a lost paradise in dreams, but they are also harsh and uncompromising places. If you dream of reaching an oasis in the desert, you are probably dreaming of having sex after a long spell of abstinence. The oasis, with its fringe of palm trees and its central pool of water, sometimes symbolizes your sexual organs.

Dildo

The dildo, or artificial penis, has many of the same dream qualities as the banana. If you dream you are making love to someone with a dildo attached to your body, you are possibly expressing your feelings that you want to continue your sexual relationship with them, but not in a very committed way. If *they* are making love to *you* with a dildo, then you may subconsciously think that behind their apparent affection, they are insincere about their sexual feelings. Dildos can take many forms in your erotic dreams. Since relatively few women have actually seen one or used one, anything that performs the same function as a dildo can be brought into your dream as a dildo image. Bananas, cucumbers, bottles, or rolling pins. In this excerpt a 35-year-old New Rochelle housewife dreams of something most original:

I was dancing across a polished ballroom, under a whole glittering galaxy of chandeliers. I was dancing with the man who had come from our real estate people to value the house. I thought he was good-looking when he arrived, and he'd been around a couple of times for coffee, and I'd already started to wonder if we might go to bed together. Now, here I was, dancing around with him in my dream. He was dressed in a shiny red suit, and I was wearing a jewel-encrusted ballgown that was completely topless. But I was wearing diamonds and sapphires in necklaces on my breasts, and my hair was studded with jewels. As we danced, the man from the real estate corporation said that he'd always liked me from the moment he first saw me, and there was nothing in the world he wanted to do more than give me pleasure. I felt breathless, just the way I always do when I'm sexually excited. But instead of taking out his cock, he produced a hero sandwich, all stuffed with salad and tomatoes and meat and pickles, and he said he was going to fuck me with that. I told him he had to be kidding. But he said no, he wanted our relationship to start off on an informal basis, and that was the way he wanted it. Well, the climax of the dream was that I bent over on the ballroom floor and touched my toes, and the real estate man hiked my gown up at the back, then he started to push the hero sandwich into my pussy. All the salad and the meat were squelching and sliding about, and there was mayonnaise and stuff streaming down my legs. The feeling was very sexy — very sensual — particularly when a whole lot of people came around and stared at me. That turned me on. But after a while, bent over there with a two-foot hero pushed up my vagina, I began to feel pretty disillusioned.

There is another quality in dildo dreams apart from showing you how much real affection your sexual relationships may lack. That's the quality of *ritual sex*, particularly ritual defloration. Worship of phallic objects goes back to the dawn of organized religion, and as late as the eighth century there were ecclesiastical edicts warning Christians not to bow down to the *fascinum*, or phallic symbol. In France, Belgium, and Italy brides would offer their virginity to a saint instead of their husband, by penetrating themselves with a wooden phallus. If you have dildo dreams in which there is a religious or ceremonial theme, then it's possible that you have unconscious desires to have sex with the man in your life in a much more meaningful way than you are at present. You believe that offering your body is important both emotionally and spiritually, and you would like him to take your offer just as seriously. There is a hint of masochism in this kind of dream, too. Men who dream of penetrating women with dildos often have a slightly sadistic streak, and derive pleasure from the humiliation the woman suffers from being violated by an inanimate object.

Dirt

Sexual dreams of dirt almost invariably show that your conscience is working overtime, and that you're worried about the moral implications of your sex life. The dirt will often appear on your clothes, and may be no more than a spot on your cuff, but you will be concerned that other people will notice it, and you may try (unsuccessfully) to wipe it off. Some sexual dreams of dirt go the whole hog, and show exactly how filthy you think sex is. Here's an excerpt from a long dream that was sent to me by an 18-year-old girl from Baltimore, Maryland:

My boyfriend John and me, we're all alone in the house. I know we're all alone, and I know that he's going to suggest we have sexual intercourse. I'm excited, but also I'm scared. I don't think I'm old enough to have regular intercourse, and I don't want to have an unwanted baby, but there's something about sex that kind of draws me to it. It seems kind of *wicked*, and that's what excites me. Anyway, in the dream, John starts to unbutton my dress, and then he takes off my bra and my panties, till I'm nude. Then he takes off his own clothes. His organ is big and hard, and I remember how it seemed to *beat*, like a pulse. He takes me by the hand and he leads me through to the bathroom. I'm absolutely stunned, because the tub is halfway full with mud. John climbs in, and I climb in too, and we kiss and roll around in this mud, until our bodies are brown and dripping. My breasts look as though they've been dipped in chocolate, and John's organ is sticking up like a brown candy bar. I even have mud in my mouth. Anyway, John gets on top of me, and he starts to make love to me. I lie back in the sloppy mud and let it cover my hair and my body. John's almost finished, almost gotten to the end of his lovemaking, when he takes his organ right out of me, and lets his come drop in the mud. He says: 'There, if you want it, there it is.' I lean forward and take a mouthful of mud and come, and I almost choke.

One woman from New York who was having an illicit affair told me that she had dream after dream of visiting the cleaners to get rid of sex stains on her clothes. If you persistently dream of dirt, it's time you sat down and thought about your sexual situation, and whether you're truly happy about it.

Dogs

Dogs are traditionally interpreted as bearers of ill luck, and the ancients warned that you could expect danger if you dreamed about them. But if a dog appears in a sexual dream, it's possible that it represents the way you feel about your current sexual relationship. If you love dogs, and you think about them as faithful and loyal companions, then that's the way you feel about your lover. But if you dislike dogs and find them untrustworthy and mean, then your relationship is obviously not going so well. If you dream that you're having intercourse with a dog, it may mean that you're physically revolted by your present lover. Or it may mean that you regard him as nothing more than an obedient animal, only good for following orders and having sex with you. There is an enormous range of dream literature about dogs, and it is impossible to go into it very deeply here. But take note of the breed of dog you have dreamed about and its color (German shepherds represent lovers who can be fiercely faithful but also passionate and dangerous; greyhounds represent lovers who are full of sexual energy, but fretful and inconstant; poodles represent loyal but ineffectual and sometimes effeminate men).

Doll

If you dream that your husband or lover is reduced to the size of a doll, his sexual status has, for some reason, been substantially diminished in your eyes. If you dream about a favorite doll of your childhood, you may be feeling regrets for your lost youth, but probably because there is some suggestion in the air that you might become a mother yourself.

Donkey

Some old-style dream books insisted that the donkey was a symbol of sexual relationships, and that if you dreamed a donkey was braying, it meant your illicit sexual activities were about to be discovered. If you have an erotic dream in which a donkey appears, it could mean that you are anxious about your sexual partner's stubbornness and apparent disinterest in you.

E

Ears

If you dream that a man is trying to have sex with you in your ear, this can mean that you are prepared to tolerate sexual intimacy with him, provided you don't have to make any emotional commitment. In other words, you are turning your head away. If you have a sexual dream in which your ear-lobes are being pierced for silver ear-rings, it's possible that you're being warned to listen again to some gossip or opinions about your lover. If the ear-rings are gold, then this may be an admonition to do just the opposite, and disregard hearsay that runs him down. Most objects placed in the ear can be considered to be messages or information.

Eating

Sexual dreams often involve food and eating, and it may help you in your interpretation to remember what you were trying to consume. I say 'trying' because many women find it difficult to eat things in their dreams and swallow them properly, just as many people find it impossible to make a successful telephone call in their dreams. If you were obviously eating something phallic, like a banana or a chicken leg, then you may have been dreaming about oral sex. But various foods have various different meanings. Eating raw eggs in a sex dream can signify swallowing semen; eating boiled eggs can signify ovulation and pregnancy; eating soft pulpy fruits may mean that you are feeling sexually self-indulgent and passionate; eating bread and cakes may mean that you're basically bored with your sexual relationship. If the food in your dream is very hot or spicey, that can show that your sexual relationship is volatile and awkward to handle, and that you're having trouble keeping it under control.

Ecstasy

In many sexual dreams, women are capable of reaching a peak of ecstasy that seems to elude them in waking life. These ecstatic dreams could mean several different things.

They could mean that you have already attained ecstasy in your sex life without realizing it; they could mean that you are capable of achieving ecstasy and should go on searching for it; or they could be an insight into an idealized feeling that you will never be able to attain. Again, it depends on the context of the dream, how you achieve ecstasy, and with whom. Here's a dream of ecstasy from a 21-year-old Los Angeles girl:

I'm dreaming that I'm floating on a huge lily pad. I'm actually inside that Victorian painting of the ondines, the water nymphs, where they're trying to pull the handsome young guy into the lily pool. I have these diaphanous robes, and my hair is all tied up with ribbons, and I feel very lazy and beautiful. Then I dream that I'm dreaming all this, and I wake up. I reach out and I feel naked skin. I open my eyes (in my dream) and there are two young men lying next to me, one on each side, and they're watching me. They're twin brothers, and they look ravishing. They have blond hair, and slim brown bodies, and long fat penises that seem to stay hard all the time. When they see that I've woken up, they start to fondle and kiss me. They take a breast each, and kiss them and lick my nipples. Then they kiss me down my sides, until they both reach my pussy. They each slip a finger inside me, and start to massage me into a state of absolute frenzy. I mean, I'm gone. I scream and scream and scream because I'm so turned-on and so happy. I arch my back, and one of the twin boys starts sucking my pussy while the other one sucks my asshole. They both push their tongues inside me, one up my pussy and the other up my ass, and they start to waggle their tongues around until I'm clutching my own breasts and I'm literally weeping with the feeling of what they're doing to me. I can almost remember what it felt like now, looking down between my legs and seeing those two tousled blond heads, and feeling their fat wet tongues going wag, wag, wag inside me. I was just going to say something to them, just about to touch them, when I woke up for real. I looked around and I was all by myself. I had such a shock. I thought I'd woken up once before, but now I'd woken up for real and the boys had gone. Have you ever felt cheated?

If you have a dream in which you find a new way of achieving ecstasy, you're looking for variety and excitement in your love life. If you have a dream in which you induce sexual ecstasy in someone else, you may be too much of a sexual giver and not enough of a sexual taker. Try and balance your erotic relationships so that you get, at the very least, what's coming to you.

Electricity

Electric shocks sometimes appear in sexual dreams as an indication of heart-stopping orgasms. You can be quite sure that if you have an erotic dream in which electricity is involved, then your present sex relationship is a spirited but dangerous one, and you are concerned that you're going to get burned.

Elixir

Women who rely on drugs of various kinds sometimes dream that they have found a drug which magically makes them sexier/more attractive/more capable of reaching orgasm. The dream of a magic potion which can instantly solve all problems is by no means a new one: ancient alchemists wasted centuries searching for the Elixir of Life, which was supposed to make all who drank it immortal. If you have dreams of this kind, you are obviously dissatisfied with your sexual situation, but you won't find any easy answers. Take the dream to mean that you *do* need some kind of way out, but that it will probably be a long and painstaking business. Most dreams compress time and space, and combine several different meanings in one image. An elixir is a simplistic way of showing you that you need to seek a viable solution to your sexual problems.

Engine

Motors and engines sometimes represent sexual intercourse itself, and its rhythmic action. Car and motorcycle
engines have strong sexual associations even in waking
life, and in dreams they appear in all kinds of erotic
contexts. This is the dream of a 17-year-old Connecticut
girl:

I dreamed I had to go into the school boiler-room to find some
walnuts. I've often passed the boiler-room door when it's open
in the summer, and seen the boilers and stuff down there, but I
never thought that I'd ever dream about it. I went down the iron
ladder and there was a huge engine there, with a fat gray cylinder
thing and lots of pipes and valves and moving parts. It was
humming and throbbing and going backwards and forwards. I
knew I had to climb over this machine if I wanted to reach the
walnuts, so I put one leg over the fat gray cylinder. I was
frightened, because the engine was making a lot of noise, and it
had such life of its own. It was hot, too, and it almost burnt my
thighs. But when I was halfway across like that, with my legs
astride it, I began to feel nice. I mean sexy nice. It was moving
backwards and forwards between my legs, and humming and
vibrating, and if I pressed myself against it, it made me feel real
good. I wasn't wearing any panties, and somehow I managed to
press my sex parts right against it, until I could feel every single
shudder go right through me. I was more and more excited, and
I knew that I was going to reach an orgasm. Then I heard
someone say: 'What about the walnuts?' and I had to jump off
the machine and pretend that nothing had happened.

Eruption

If a volcano erupts in a sexual dream, it's usually a sign
that you have powerful bottled-up passions that need
release. Earthquakes and tremors, however, can be caused
by your fears that your sexual relationship is coming apart
at the seams, and if you dream that a chasm opens beneath

your feet, you are worried that your present affair is about to split apart.

Escalator

If you dream that you are going up an escalator, and you are sexually aroused by it, then you could be dreaming of intercourse. But it may also mean that you feel your sexual ability is improving, and that you are discovering new and varied sex techniques to improve your love life.

Eunuch

Sexless men, when they appear in sexual dreams, can have several fascinating implications. If you have a dream in which you discover your would-be lover or husband-to-be is a eunuch, and you have never actually made love to him before, then you may be concerned that he is not going to satisfy your sexual appetites, and that he may be prudish in bed. Now, you don't have thoughts like this for nothing – so try and think what he may have done to give you that impression. If you dream that you are castrating him yourself, your dream may be warning you that your sexual personality is too strong for him, and that you will lose his love if you continue to dominate him so strongly. It could also mean that you are unconsciously afraid of carrying on a sexual relationship with him, and that you are trying to emasculate him before he can hurt you. Eunuchs often appear as reliable friends in highly erotic dreams because they cannot threaten you sexually, and it may be that they represent those parts of your personality which are not excited or aroused by sex.

Eyes

To dream that you are having sex while being watched by disembodied eyes is an indication that you feel guilty about what you are doing. If you dream that you look intently into your lover's eyes during sex, you may be trying to discover if he's really sincere about his feelings for you. If you try to cover his eyes in a sexual way (e.g. by kissing them, licking them, or gluing them together with sexual fluids) then you may feel that he doesn't love you any more, but you're trying to delay his recognition of that fact. If you dream that your lover ejaculates his semen into your eyes, it's possible that you feel blinded by your sexual desire for him, although I have come across dreams in which women have said their vision was improved and clarified by having semen in their eyes. This may be related to the primitive belief that semen has magical properties, since most of the women who reported dreams like these were nearsighted. Animal eyes (particularly green ones) are an indication of lust or jealousy. Blue, wide-open eyes are symbolic of honesty and faithfulness. According to one old dream book, if you made love to a man with violently crossed eyes, you were going to marry a rich husband!

F

Fat

Sexual dreams of fatness are often dreams of pregnancy, but they can also mean that you are worried about your weight. Most women have to diet every now and again to retain their sexual attractiveness to men. If you dream that you are very fat and bloated because you are full of gas or wind, this may mean that you feel your personal vanity and self-esteem will be found out by the man you love, and that you will be humiliated because of it. If you are very fat and heavy in your dream, you could be feeling that the responsibility of your present sexual relationship is too much for you. A sexual dream of fatness could also be evoked by your forthcoming period.

Fire

In erotic dreams fire almost always represents passion and lust. There is probably an indication that you are more interested in oral sex than any other variations if you persistently dream of fire in a sexual context, because fire has such oral associations – fire 'licks' and fire 'devours'. You talk of 'hot' kisses and 'fiery' words. Susanne K. Langer, in her book on philosophy and symbolism, made the point that 'fire is a natural symbol of life and passion, though it is the one element in which nothing can actually live.' Fire is destructive, and when you have a relationship of great heat and intensity, it can destroy your love as quickly as it builds it up. If you have a sexual dream of uncontrolled fire, you are probably relishing the passion of your present sexual relationship, but you are aware that it cannot last for ever. If you see the fire in a hearth or a barbecue, under rigid control, then you are dreaming about domestic love – regular sexual intercourse in its 'proper place'. If you dream about trying a light a fire, perhaps by striking matches or rubbing two sticks together, you are trying to spark sexual interest in a man you like, or trying to rekindle desire in a man who has grown indifferent. If you have a sexual dream of charred and smoking ruins, then you are admitting to yourself that your love has finally burned itself out.

I was making love to Harry in a big bed with curtains. I was lying back, and I was loving every minute of it, every gorgeous stroke of his pecker. I clung on to his shoulders, and I twisted my hips, and I kissed him and told him I loved him. He didn't answer. I looked up at his handsome face, and I felt his pecker sliding in and out of me, and I said: 'This won't be the last time, will it?' He didn't say a word, although he did smile. He came, and I came too, and it spread over me like a warm sun. I put my arms around him to hug him, and I found that I was hugging a heap of papery ashes, and nothing else.

Fish

Even though fish have a phallic shape, their appearance in erotic dreams is usually mysterious and hard to explain. They rarely seem to be seen in an easily understandable context, and this leads me to believe that they often represent the more mystic side of sex. Fish are cold and alien and remote, and it's possible that they enter your erotic dreams as a reminder of the intellectual and spiritual aspects of human relationships. Folklore regards fish as 'brain-food', and symbolically fish have powerful Christian connotations. Fish may also represent feelings of frigidity and revulsion that you have for some sexual partner.

Flowers

In many erotic dreams, flowers represent your female sexual organs. They also have traditional symbolic meanings, and it's possible that particular flowers, when they appear in your sexual dreams, may hold similar implications. Broken flowers represent lost virginity; roses represent fresh and passionate women; lilies represent purity and virginity; dried flowers represent spinsterhood; daisies represent youth and innocence; heavily scented flowers represent sensuality, but also betrayal and deception. Circular flowers are sometimes supposed to symbolize the womb, or the circle of life and fate. Dead flowers represent withered hopes, and the end of sexual affairs, but they also have their optimistic side to them. When one bunch of flowers is dead, it's quite possible to go out and pick a fresh spray, and start again.

Flying

Erotic dreams of flying — unlike ordinary dreams of flying — are mainly concerned with sexual skill. If you are trying to fly in your sexual dream, then you are striving for better erotic abilities, and your flying dexterity will give you a pretty clear indication of how good you think your bed-time technique really is. If you fly shakily or upside down, then you're probably worried that your sexual skill leaves something to be desired. But if you soar and glide with ease, you're quite confident that your loving is up to scratch. If you dream that you're flying on your own, at a great altitude, then you may think that you're entitled to be haughty and aloof about your sexual relationships. If you dream that you're flying, but you crash to the ground, then you're anxious about how long your current sexual relationship is going to continue. Here's an erotic dream of flying in which a 29-year-old New York woman began to discover how nervous she was about her marriage:

I'm light, I can't keep my feet on the ground. I'm trying to walk around my apartment, but I'm so light and floaty that I can only manage to touch the floor once in every four or five steps. Then I'm so light that I can't get down to the floor at all. Bob opens the living-room door, and he lets a howling wind come in. My skirt is blown right up, and I'm only wearing tights underneath. He sort of floats through the room and seizes my ankle. Then he comes nearer by pulling himself up along my legs. He starts shouting at me, asking me what the hell's going on. The wind is so strong that I can hardly hear him. I say that I'm floating around, and I'm not sure how long I'll be able to stay here in this apartment, because any moment now the wind's going to blow me away. Bob nods as if he understands what I'm saying, then he struggles out of his clothes and lets them scatter all over the room. The wind is even stronger, and I have to press my hands against the ceiling. Bob floats around me, and I try to kiss his cock as it drifts past my face, but I miss. Then he floats around so that he can make love to me from behind. He puts his arms around me, and starts to push his cock in between my legs, but of course I'm still wearing tights and he can't get in. He tugs my tights right down, but as soon as he gets them right off, the wind catches me and I blow away. I float through a tiny crack in the window, and I'm so frightened that I wake up.

This dream of flying (or floating) indicated that the woman was unsure of her sexual abilities. She was trying her best to control her technique, but in the face of her husband's strong desires (the wind) she was powerless. She even forgot to remove her tights before making love, and the embarrassment she felt at that piece of sexual incompetence blew her straight out of her husband's apartment. She had many dreams of a similar nature, and it was only when she was able to admit her fears, and seek her husband's reassurance and help, that she stopped having them.

Fruit

When fruit appears in your sexual dreams – and particularly when you're eating it – you can be fairly certain that it represents the sexual organs. Bananas we've already talked about. Apples and pears sometimes symbolize the breasts or the testicles. Peaches and figs and fruits with clefts in them represent female sexual organs. If you have an erotic dream in which you are stealing fruit, or trying to eat fruit in secrecy, you may be feeling unconsciously ashamed of your sexual feelings. If you have a dream in which you discover that the fruit you want to eat is overripe or rotten, then your dream is probably telling you that your sexual relationship is in the same condition. To dream of strange, unknown fruit is to dream of sexual deviations that you would like to try.

Fuck

Although you may never use obscene language in waking life, your dreaming mind is not so polite. Many women have told me that they have been shocked and surprised by the language they have used in their sexual dreams, and even by the words in which they have described the dream to themselves in their own minds when they have woken up. As one Cincinnati woman said: 'I knew what the word "cunt" meant, of course. But I would never use it. In my dream, though, I imagined that a man was looking at my "cunt". That was the way my brain kind of described it when I was asleep, and that's the only way I can talk about it now. Thinking of my private parts as a "cunt" gave the dream a thrill which I can't conjure up without using that word.' When you have an erotic dream full of 'dirty words', it may indicate that you feel that sex is 'naughty but nice', and that you are trying to recapture some of the forbidden thrill it had for you when you were younger. Even though words like 'fuck' and 'cunt' have a long and respectable etymology, they are used today for the deliberate purpose of shocking or stimulating (or both) and when you use them in your sexual dreams you are using them for precisely this reason. Occasionally, words will appear in your erotic dreams that seem obscene in the dream, but which are quite innocuous in reality. One girl told me she dreamed she was masturbating — an activity she described as 'huddling'. The word seemed so vulgar in the dream that she felt ashamed to think of it. It's an interesting illustration of the fact that words, and dreams, are exactly what you make of them.

G

Games

When you have erotic dreams that feature games – dice or chess or backgammon or Monopoly – you are usually dreaming about sexual competitiveness. Are you vying with another woman for the attentions of the same man? Are you competing *against* your lover, rather than making love *with* him? Whatever the game, you feel there are problems in your sexual relationship which need to be solved. It may help you if you can recall what kind of game you were playing in the dream, and what the state of the game was when the dream ended. One woman was able to make a sketch of a game of chess she was playing with her husband, and from the position of the players it seemed that she felt her husband was trying to outwit and deceive her. Ball games and athletic games very often represent the sexual act in dreams. Sometimes, your dreaming mind will invent a game that sums up your sexual situation for you:

This was an indoor game. We were playing it in a place that looked like a community hall, or a school gymnasium. I knew my husband was playing, as well as me, but there were lots of other people there that I knew. There were two lines of people, and they stood facing each other over thirty or forty yards. Each line was made up of men and women alternately. We were all naked, except for white baseball boots. I wasn't sure how the game started. There was some sort of silent gong that only dogs could hear. What we had to do was run across to the man or woman on the other side of the hall, have sex with them until we reached a climax, then everyone crossed over and did the same thing to someone else. The first person to have a climax with everyone else was going to be the winner. I rushed across as quick as I could. My next-door neighbor was there, Ted Cohen. He said: 'Quick, quick, you have to do it.' His penis was big and awkward. We had to have intercourse standing up. He lifted me up, and he didn't seem strong enough to hold me, but he managed to push his penis into me, and bounce me up and down on his thighs. I kept my eyes tight shut and tried to think about having a climax. I didn't think I was going to be able to make it. I opened my eyes again, and I saw Gary, my husband, having intercourse with the brunette girl from across the road. She had huge breasts, and Gary really seemed to be enjoying himself. Just for that, I jumped up and down even faster on Ted Cohen's penis, until we both came. I was jealous, but I was going to show him if it was the last thing I did. I ran across to the brunette girl, and I had to have sex with her. Go down on her, you know. There was semen running out of her vagina, and she tried to stop it with her hand. I said: 'What's wrong with you? That's my husband's semen you're hiding in there. If I'm not entitled to it, I don't know who the hell is.'

This was part of a much longer dream from a 29-year-old housewife from New Jersey. The dream was describing, in visual terms, her suspicions that her husband was growing interested in swinging. He had started to mention it to her, and ask her views about it. Her dream turned it into a ritualized game, and showed her very clearly that she ought to stay away from it. Jealousy and swinging don't mix and match. If you have erotic dreams in which you're faced with confusing and complicated games to play, it may be that you feel unsure of your physical and emotional ability to continue your present sexual relationship. If you dream that you're playing for money (one-armed bandits, chemin-de-fer) then you could be dreaming about difficulties in reaching orgasm. If you dream that you're always watching games, rather than participating, then your dream is warning you not to keep yourself aloof and apart from sexual involvement.

Gardens

Some ancient dream interpreters believed that gardens represented the female sexual organs, and there is some evidence that bushes and shrubs and flowers occasionally symbolize pubic hair. But, more often, an erotic dream which features a garden seems to be showing you how you unconsciously feel about your present sexual relationship. If the garden is neat and tidy, with clipped hedges and trim borders, you may feel that your relationship is controlled and orderly. If the garden is wild and beautiful, you may feel that your relationship is just the same. Some women have had repeated dreams about a garden, and have watched it die and deteriorate just as their sexual relationship has died and deteriorated. Remember that gardens are arranged and maintained by people, and that they are highly symbolic of life and what you are prepared to make of it. For more detailed interpretations, see *1,001 Erotic Dreams Interpreted*.

Gates

Dreams of closed and locked gates, when they appear in a sexual context, can mean that you feel trapped and stagnant in your sexual life. They can also signify your unwillingness to have intercourse with a particular man. If the gates are open, and you're going through them, you're dreaming of broadening your sexual horizons, and you may be prepared to commit your body to new erotic experiences.

Gestures

If you are the kind of woman who is reserved about sex and sexual activities, you may have erotic dreams in which blatantly sexual gestures are disguised by rather politer activities. If you are sewing, by hand or by machine, you could be dreaming of masturbation. If you are rocking backwards and forwards, in a chair or on a ship or bus, you could be dreaming of sexual intercourse.

Grandparents

If your grandparents appear in a sexual dream, they may represent the security that you feel your present relationship lacks. Fathers and mothers very rarely appear as figures of protection and succor. They have been too close to you in your sexual development to have the benevolent remoteness of grandparents. If you dream of a dead grandparent, you may be trying to solve a sexual problem in your relationship, since dead grandparents often seem to appear with advice or news.

Gum

Chewing gum in a sexual dream is sometimes symbolic of fellatio. Porno actress Emily Smith, from San Francisco, attests that male sperm, if you hold it in your mouth for some minutes, can be chewed and pulled into long strings like gum. If you are chewing gum in your dream while you are actually having sex, you may feel too casual about your current sexual affairs. If your lover is chewing gum, you may feel that he is too offhand with you.

Guns

In a society so acclimatized to the use of handguns as America, it is inevitable that they should drift into your dreams as symbols of the male penis. They are hard, aggressive, and they shoot out bullets. They have masculine power. It could be interesting to compare the frequency of erotic dreams about guns dreamed by American women with similar sexual dreams dreamed by British women, who have no daily awareness of guns in their society. That wouldn't mean that British women dream about penises any the less. Among the primitive Australian tribe of the Yir Yoront, where guns are completely unknown, they dream of penises stretching for miles from a man to a woman. If you have erotic dreams in which a male is pointing a gun at you, or shooting a gun at you, take careful note of how you respond to his action in the dream. It could tell you a great deal about your feelings for him. As an example, here's a handgun dream from a 33-year-old Baltimore woman:

I was standing behind the cocktail bar where I work some evenings, and I was wiping glasses. It seemed so natural and real that I didn't even think it was a dream. Then my boyfriend came in through the door. He was smiling, although I didn't know why. Because it was him, I unbuttoned my blouse and I bared my breasts. He sat at the counter and looked me up and down. He was smiling all the while. Then he pointed something at me, and I looked and saw a pistol in his hand. It was a dark red color, and I could see the hole where the bullets came out. I asked him if he was going to shoot me. He said: 'Don't be the stupid skating rink.' I held my breasts in my hands, and he shot me in the breasts. It felt exciting. I was surprised that it didn't hurt me at all. I raised my dress, and he shot me again, three or four times, in the stomach and the cunt. I dropped to the floor, and I was lying there feeling faint. I thought: 'Now I'm dying.' But down there, I knew I could masturbate without my boyfriend or any of the customers seeing me. So I put my hand inside my panties, and I masturbated and masturbated until I finally came. Then my boyfriend looked over the counter and said: 'How was I?'

This woman had been having an on-and-off affair for two years with a man whom she didn't count as a great lover. She saw his penis as a gun because she always considered he was remote and unemotional, and that's just what a handgun is. It fucks from afar. The reason she dropped out of sight and masturbated under the counter was that she always had to stimulate herself to orgasm after her boyfriend had made love to her. He never brought her off himself. So, if you have erotic dreams about guns, remember that you're possibly dreaming of penises, but also remember that they're penises with the same qualities as guns — they're used from a distance. If you have an erotic dream in which you're firing a gun, it may mean that you're impatient to take control of a sexual relationship yourself, and be the dominant partner.

H

Hair

Hair is one of the most fascinating and multifarious of sexual dream images. It has always had sexual associations (Samson's virility was stored in his hair; Rapunzel's hair was a ladder for her lover; and the eighteenth-century poet Alexander Pope knew exactly what he was talking about in his tale of a stolen curl, *The Rape of the Lock*). If you dream that you have very long hair, you are probably dreaming of your femininity and fertility, but if you dream that you are hiding your nudity behind your long hair, then you have serious doubts about your sexual attractiveness. In sexual dreams, hair can sometimes represent a visible manifestation of the ideas that are going on in someone's head. The Cambodians thought they could dispose of unwelcome nightmares by cutting their hair off. If you dream that your lover has very long hair, you are not dreaming that he is effeminate; in fact, you're probably dreaming the exact opposite. If you become tangled in that long hair, then his sexuality is involving and enmeshing you. If his hair is actually choking you, then the intensity of your sexual relationship is too much for you to handle. If you have erotic dreams in which your hair is falling out, then you are dreaming of your fears of losing your lover. Is this a fear without foundation, or have you unconsciously assimilated some information that has provoked you into having that dream? Hair is a crown, it is a means of self-identification. Apart from the fact that he died at the Little Big Horn, all that most people remember about General Custer was his long yellow hair. Then there were the Beatles – 'the Mersey moptops'. And Jimi Hendrix. When you have a sexual dream in which you have a distinctive or elaborate hairstyle, you are probably dreaming about your womanly individuality, your own sexual specialness. In this dream excerpt, a 38-year-old Chicago woman explains what she felt about her hair:

I was walking along North Michigan Avenue on a breezy summer's day and I was attracting all kinds of attention because I was wearing nothing but small salmon-pink panties, and the hugest coiffure you've ever seen. I could see myself in mirrors and store windows as I walked along the sidewalk. My hair was piled up into layers and layers of soft brown curls, a huge hairy ball on top of my head, and all the hair was decorated with butterflies and combs – then it fell down over my shoulders in a huge cape made out of curly hair, and halfway down my back. I felt beautiful, and I walked with a very straight back, and I really strutted along. Standing by the corner was a cab driver. He was just like one of those toothy handsome men you see in *Viva* or something. He was wearing a peaked cap, and blue jeans so tight that you could see his hard rod sticking halfway down his leg. He took my arm, and he guided me over to his cab. It was a weird kind of cab, covered in some kind of orange leather. Then he pulled down my panties, while a whole crowd of people were watching, and he said: 'This here's the Queen of the Bay!' I posed and stuck my butt out, and I could see myself in a mirror across the street, with my huge curly hair. My body was real smooth and curvy, like a Vargas girl. The cab driver dropped his jeans. He had lovely muscly legs, and a big meaty piece. He buried his hands in my hair, and clung on to it while he forced his piece into my pussy. I looked down to see him going into me, and I couldn't believe it when I saw that my pubic hair was all thick and curly as well.

There are other important images in this dream – particularly the mirrors – but the huge curly hairstyle is an outstanding symbol of sexual self-confidence and even vanity. There is nothing embarrassed or hesitant about the way this woman felt about sex. She knew what she had to offer, she knew what she wanted, and she knew what she was prepared to do to get it. If you have dreams about losing your pubic hair, you are possibly anxious about losing your sexual attractiveness. If your lover loses his pubic hair, you may be worried that he's being unfaithful to you. But if you have erotic dreams of shaving each other's pubic hair, you may be dreaming about a new closeness and intimacy between you. If you have sexual dreams of kissing a bearded man, there may be some elements of bisexuality in your make-up, since beards are so strongly reminiscent of female genitalia. One slang term for intercourse is 'piercing the bearded clam'. If you have a sexual dream in which you cut or crop your hair, you may be dreaming that you want to make a fresh start in your sexual life. You have been too sexually self-indulgent, and you feel it's time to put your energies into other aspects of life.

Hats

Hats, like hair, are often symbols of authority or individuality. They sometimes appear in dreams to show that whoever is wearing them wants to conceal their thoughts or intentions (this is logical, since hair sometimes represents ideas and thoughts). Important people in your sexual dreams will frequently wear important hats – crowns, helmets, and so on. If you have an erotic dream in which you are making love with your hat on, then you are dreaming that your sexual relationship is not permanent, and that you are not prepared to commit yourself to it fully. 'Anywhere I hang my hat is home,' says the song, and you are obviously not going to do that. If you have a dream in which your hat is too large for you, you are worried that you are unable to cope with the emotional demands of your sex life. If your hat is too small, then you are feeling repressed by your lover's lack of deep emotion and intellectual capacity. Hats with plumes or feathers in them can represent sexual exhibitionism, but they also have a traditional interpretation of mourning and ill fortune.

Homosexuality

Many dreams of homosexuality are, in reality, dreams of self-love. In a dream, everything and anything is possible, so you can become two people and make love to yourself.

I dreamed I was lying in bed. I know it was my bed, because it had the same candy-striped sheets. There was a naked girl lying asleep next to me. I reached out and touched her breasts. They felt wonderful – warm and soft, with big nipples. I climbed on top of the girl, and I kissed her and told her that I loved her. I kissed her lips and her neck, and then I moved down and kissed her breasts and her stomach. I felt my heart beating, and I knew exactly what I was going to do next. I pushed her thighs apart, and there was her vagina, all hot from being asleep. I scooped my hands under her bottom, and I raised her hips towards me, and I plunged my face right into that hot, juicy vagina, and kissed it and licked it and sucked it. Then something made me look up, towards the girl's face. I had a feeling like dropping down too fast in an elevator. I mean, I felt *scared* – because the girl was me.

There was no need to feel scared. What she was dreaming about was no more outrageous than masturbation. But what if the girl you're making love to is somebody else? Again, there's no need to be unduly disturbed unless you're already conscious of lesbian tendencies. In every one of us, there's a mish-mosh of sexual characteristics, both hetero-sexual and homosexual. During waking life, we keep our less conventional sexual tastes firmly repressed, but during sleep they can have free rein. If you have dreams in which your lover or husband is making love to another man, you don't necessarily suspect his virility. More likely, you're feeling jealous because you think that his relationships with men are strong and loyal, and that because you're a woman, you're excluded from them.

Horse

Horses, especially stallions, can represent proud, virile sexual characteristics. If you have a sexual dream about wild horses, then you may be dreaming about uncontrolled sexual emotions, or your fears that your lover is too independent and self-willed to be kept in your bed for very long. Some dream interpretations suggest that if you are kicked in the stomach by a horse, then you have a desire to be taken by an ardent and passionate lover. Black horses represent unruly passions; white horses represent death; brown horses represent devotion and loyalty. If you dream that you are riding a horse, and deriving sexual pleasure from it, you feel that you have your mate firmly under your thumb as far as sex is concerned.

House

Houses can either represent someone you know, with windows for eyes and a front door for a mouth, or — more commonly — they can represent your sexual relationship. If you have a sexual dream in which a house figures prominently, then take a close look through your memory at the rooms you saw and what condition they were in. Cold, bleak houses are symbolic of cold and indifferent sexual relationships. Warm, cozy houses full of fur and beds are symbolic of passionate, close relationships.

I dreamed that we had rented a little summer cottage. It was hard work squeezing in through the door, but once we'd gotten inside, it was dark and warm and lovely. We took off all our clothes, and had intercourse in the darkness. Mike's body felt wonderful — soft and smooth like it always does. I held his penis in my hand and took him through the house and up the stairs. But when I opened the bedroom door, I stopped. There was another woman lying on the bed. She was naked — a redhead with big breasts and a pearl necklace. She said something to me in a harsh voice, but I ran out, and got away as fast as I could.

This — the dream of a 24-year-old Boston girl — is expressing a deep subconscious fear that her fiance had another woman on his mind. Downstairs, in the dark, their relationship was fine, but upstairs, in his brain, she suspected that an old flame still lurked. I think it's interesting how the 'old flame' (her own words) is translated into a red-hot redhead. Take most dream houses to stand for the structure of your sex life as a whole, unless the house is familiar and unimportant in your dream, in which case it is nothing more than a piece of convenient scenery against which your mind can play out its sexual dramas.

I

Impotence

If you have a sexual dream in which your lover appears to be impotent, you may be concerned that he no longer finds you attractive. The meaning will often depend on the mood of the dream. If the impotence is rather humorous and silly(if his penis bends like rubber and you are both laughing about it), then there is nothing to worry about – it is simply a light-hearted dream in which serious achievements become ludicrously impossible. But if there is anxiety and disappointment in the dream – if you were desperately hoping that he would be able to have sex with you, and you are shattered by his inability to do so – then you may have problems on your hands.

Incest

Despite the complexity of interpretation that Freud and Jung brought to sexual dreams of incest – father-figures and mother-figures and all the rest of the symbols and archetypes – it is plain that many women dream of intercourse with their fathers or brothers for very straightforward reasons. They have always been aware of their fathers' or brothers' maleness, and in dreams, where morality is not as demanding as it is in waking life, they can explore that maleness by making love to them. Sometimes the dream will be haunted by conscientious objections, but as Dr Ann Faraday noticed, most people have no qualms about sex with their relatives when they're dreaming. So even if you don't like the idea of dreaming about your father or your brother, don't get too anxious about it. It's no worse than dreaming about sex with anyone else.

I was doing a strip in front of my whole family – my father, my mother, my older sister and my brother. I was standing on the dining-room table peeling off my clothes one by one to the sound of this crude stripper-type music. I kicked off my shoes, peeled off my dress, undid my bra and danced up and down the table in nothing but panties. Then I stood in front of my father, licking my lips and slowly, slowly pulling my panties down, until

I was nude. I struck a saucy legs-apart pose in front of him, and said: 'There – how about that?' Everyone clapped. I thought I was really clever. Father stood up and hung his coat over the back of the chair. He took off his suspenders, dropped his pants, and sat down on one of the chairs around the table. I looked down and his cock was poking up between his shirt-tails. He held a hand up and said: 'Come on, Sarah, come and sit down on your old pa's lap.' I opened my legs and jumped. I seemed to float down. Father held my hands, and guided me down as I floated. His cock went into me like two spaceships docking in space. I sat on his cock, with my legs still wide apart, and I looked into his face, and I thought: 'So this is what it's like to fuck your own father. It's just ordinary!'

That was the dream of a 19-year-old Seattle girl. She was going through a difficult time with her boyfriend when she dreamed it, and she may have been trying to find sexual security within her own family. But there was certainly nothing disturbed about her, and when she woke up she felt no sexual attraction for her father whatsoever.

Incubus

An incubus, according to medieval churchmen, was a demon in male form who spent most of his nights creeping into the bedchambers of sleeping women and forcing them to have intercourse. In 1494, the theologian Bartolomeo de Spina said that some incubi were formed 'from the odor of men and women in intercourse.' According to another theologian, incubi took from young men semen that was 'abundant, very thick, very warm and rich in spirits' and transferred it to sleeping women. Although dreams of being raped by evil spirits have declined since medieval times, some women still have nightmares in which they are assaulted by strangers or monsters while they sleep. Often, women dream these dreams when they are feeling sexually frustrated. They feel like intercourse, but they are not prepared to take the responsibility for initiating a casual act of sex. Therefore, they dream that a mysterious stranger has entered their room and taken the responsibility off their shoulders.

I dreamed that my door opened, and there was a shadowy figure standing in the doorway. He looked like The Exorcist or Orson Welles. He was dressed in black and he wore a big hat and a big cloak. He came across the room and his cloak spread over me. I couldn't see his face. He was enormously strong, and there was nothing I could do to stop him. In any case, I was paralyzed with a strange sort of fascination. I felt him tear open my nightdress from top to bottom, and I could even feel the cold night air on my bare skin. Then I felt something hard and round pushing against my vagina, like a doorknob, and I realized he was forcing his penis into me. It was too big, his penis, and I cried out, but he breathed cold breath on me, and I was completely silent. He had intercourse with me in an odd, offbeat rhythm. There was something about it that was impossible to resist. I was afraid his come was going to be black, like tar, and I was going to give birth to some awful hairy dwarf or something.

That was the sexual dream of a 36-year-old San Francisco woman who had been separated from her husband for two years. It is interesting how a medieval concept (the demonic visitor in the night) has taken on modern clothes (The Exorcist or Orson Welles). Dreams change according to social fashion and historic development, and even though their themes may be primitive, their imagery is always up-to-date.

Infection

To dream of catching an infection in a sexual dream is almost invariably an expression of anxiety about becoming pregnant. If you catch a venereal disease, you may be concerned about the consequences of your latest sexual liaison – particularly that other people may find out about it. One Los Angeles girl dreamed that her vagina developed a cold (this was after she had made love to her boyfriend in the open air), and that it kept sneezing and sniffling under her dress.

Insects

Whenever insects and bugs appear in erotic dreams, they represent some element of doubt and fear in your sex life. Insects are cold-blooded and alien. They have no conscience and they are totally cruel. If you have a sexual dream in which you are being bitten by bugs or carried off by giant ants, you are displaying deep-down masochistic tendencies, because the essence of masochistic excitement is that you have no control over your sexual fate whatsoever. There is a well-remembered scene in the strip cartoon *Phoebe Zeitgeist*, an exaggerated satire on a sadomasochistic theme, where our heroine is chained to a cave floor and voracious insects crawl all over her nude body. If the insects in your dreams are neutral or harmless, they may represent the intellectual side of your sexual relationships. If you dream that you have been bitten by insects, your sleeping mind may be trying to remind you of something important in your sex life that you ought to consider closely, but which you've overlooked. Spiders are generally symbolic of women, and their webs represent the snare of domesticity. Moths represent sexual fear and uncertainty. Butterflies symbolize beauty, but usually mental beauty rather than physical beauty – in Greek mythology, the soul was represented by Psyche, who flew with butterfly wings. Bees represent people who are drunk with love and passion. These are all ancient and dogmatic interpretations, but they may help you to understand your own sexual dreams of insects.

J

Jewels

Sexual dreams which include images of jewelry are quite common. The jewels can have many different meanings, according to the ways in which the jewelry is worn, what different jewels you find personally attractive, and whether you feel in your dream that the jewels are valuable. To discover that a jewel is made of glass is an indication that you are worried about the worth of your sexual relationship. If you see valuable and beautiful jewelry being dropped in dirt or mud ('pearls before swine') then you may be dreaming that you have given your body to someone who doesn't appreciate your sexual value. Jewels can sometimes represent a woman's sexual organs — at other times they can represent drops of precious semen. If you dream that a man you love is giving you jewelry, then you may have a desire to commit yourself to him, sexually and intellectually. There used to be a medieval game in which you tried to identify any precious stones that mysterious strangers might give you in your dreams, and then tallied the stones against whatever birth-signs they represented to discover who your future husband might be. If you were given a garnet, for instance, you would marry a Capricorn. I mention this game because it's amusing, but it can never help you identify your spouse-to-be for real.

Journeys

When you have sexual dreams which involve journeys, you may be dreaming about the progress of your entire sexual relationship, or about the progress of one sexual act. Journeys do not mean that you want to escape from your present existence. After all, the very definition of a journey is 'a traveling from one place to another'. When you journey, you expect to arrive someplace. When you escape, you don't care where you go as long as it's not where you escaped from. An erotic dream journey is often a review of your sexual relationship as far as it's progressed up to date. Your imagination may predict the course of the journey further along into the future, which always makes for interesting dreaming, but you must never accept that predicted possibilities are hard-and-fast events that will actually happen. How you interpret your dream journeys will depend on where you think you're headed, and how you're traveling. As Dr Ann Faraday points out, 'vehicles often indicate the direction in which a relationship is going' — and she cites the case of a man who dreamed he was riding on a tram in the wrong direction because he felt his wife was taking their marriage toward the wrong direction. If you have dreams of luxury travel, then you are quite content with your sexual relationship, and you feel you are making the most of it. If you dream that you are going second-class, however, you may have doubts about what you're doing, and you may be thinking that your sex partner could show his love more generously. Sometimes, a dream journey will start off well and gradually drift off course, or get caught up in a violent storm. Interpret these events straightforwardly, for they mean just what you think they mean. Your sexual relationship is drifting, or else you're involved in tension and arguments. Just as some relationships are romantic, some journeys are romantic. Here's an example from a 23-year-old student from Memphis, Tennessee:

I'm driving through an endless orchard in a kind of car. It's not like an ordinary car at all. It has one huge decorated wheel, painted with gold and blue, and then a carriage at the side which seems to hold the engine. There are several seats, all at different levels, attached to the wheel and the engine carriage on long, upcurving springs. At first, I'm driving this car by myself, and I'm traveling quickly through the orchards, not knowing what's happened or where I'm going.

Then my boyfriend Craig climbs aboard, and he takes hold of some silver and gold handles, and starts to control the car. I feel safer now. The sky has grown darker in the distance, but I don't worry too much about that. If it rains, I'm sure that Craig will think of some way to keep us dry.

He climbs up to a higher seat, quite close to mine, and I see that he's wearing his brown leather jacket but no pants at all. His dick is standing up, and much bigger than I've ever seen it. He calls me over to his seat, and I have to hold on to different strings and wires to make my way across. At last I get there, and Craig gets me to lie back in a big net, like a huge lacrosse cradle, and he buckles my legs to the sides of it with leather buckles. When he's done that, he kneels in the net between my legs and starts to finger me. I can't move my arms and legs, but he's really getting me going. When he holds his dick in his hand and gets ready to stick it in me, I'm calling out for him to *do it, do it*. I love him so much and I want him. I tell him I love him over and over. His dick I love, and his gorgeous face, and every single part of him.

He holds on to the net, and he starts to make love to me, swinging and swaying in the net. I can hear myself panting for breath. I can look and see his dick pumping into me. But before anything happens, it starts to rain very hard. The rain falls on the car's engine, and it stops. The car rolls to a standstill, and just kind of stays there in the orchard, hissing and not moving. The rain's falling real heavy, and it's running down my face and my bare body and everyplace. I look at Craig and I ask him what we ought to do. He just says: 'How should I know? I'm getting out of here!' and he climbs down and runs away through the trees. I start to cry, and I know that I'll never catch up with him now.

If you have a dream in which you miss a bus or train, then you may be feeling that you're missing out on some sexual excitement in your life. If you dream that you're riding on a bus and you don't have the money to pay your fare, you may be dreaming that you can't cope with all the demands that your sex life is making on you. In dreams where your ship can't quite get into harbor, or your plane can't land because of fog, or you can't find the street that you're headed for, you may be feeling confused and frustrated about what's going to happen in the future of your relationship.

K

Key

Sexual dreams in which keys are being pushed into locks are frequently dreams of intercourse, but there is some suggestion that the woman (possibly you yourself) is taking part in the sexual act with some reluctance. If you have a sexual dream in which you find a key, you may feel that you've at last found the answer to your sexual dissatisfaction. I recently came across a French drawing which shows a medieval woman wearing a chastity belt, gazing in amazement at a lusty-looking knight, whose penis is in the shape of a key. And a Louisiana woman told me she had had a dream in which she and her lover were locked in a prison, only to find that her lover's rigid penis was able to open all the doors.

Killing

Like many dream actions, killing someone doesn't necessarily mean that you really want to slay them, or that you hate them enough to do it. In a sexual dream, killing your lover is usually a convenient way of ending your relationship, or punishing him for things that you think he has done wrong. It shows that you're feeling aggressive and frustrated, and that you're seeking a quick and dramatic end to your sexual problems.

I met Philip on the street corner. It was raining, and we both wore raincoats. I knew that we were both naked under our raincoats, and that we were going to the docks to make love. We walked through the puddles and across the wharf until we came to a pier. We looked around to make sure that no one was watching, and then we ducked under the pier. It was quite dark under there, and it was surprisingly warm and dry. I stood against one of the upright supports and loosened my raincoat belt. It fell open, and I said to Philip: 'Look, I'm naked under this.' He stepped over and he put his hands on my breasts. I remember that his hands were cold, like ice, as if he was already dead, and my nipples went very hard because of it. He opened his own coat and his cock was raring to go. He kissed me and caressed me, and began to thrust his cock up me. We had to stop for a moment, because I thought I heard someone walking on the pier up above us, someone whistling *Sealed with a Kiss*. When they'd gone away, we started making love again, slow and quiet at first, but soon we were doing it real quick. I was aroused so much that I was biting Philip's neck, but I knew all along that we couldn't stay together, and that I was going to have to do something about it. I reached in my raincoat pocket and took out a long pair of scissors that used to belong to my mother. I reached around behind him, and opened them up, and then I pushed one blade right up his asshole. He didn't seem to notice. I started cutting with the scissors, and I cut him up into pieces. It was like cutting pastry. There wasn't any blood that I can remember. When I'd finished, I looked down on the boards of the pier to make sure I hadn't left any clues behind, and there was his cut-off cock. I picked it up and slipped it into my pocket. After all, I thought – I might need it again sometime.

That was the dream of a young San Franciscan girl whose relationship with her boyfriend was only hanging by a thread. That thread was their spasmodic sexual need for each other, and apart from that, they were indifferent and unsuited. The girl was dreaming that she was finally getting rid of Philip – although even after she'd murdered him, she was reluctant to let his penis go. She didn't feel any genuine homicidal tendencies towards him, but dreams will often interpret a broken relationship as death. After all, you will never see your unwanted lover again, and he might just as well be dead. If you dream that you're killing another woman, you may be trying to dispose of a sexual rival – but you may also be trying to destroy another manifestation of yourself, a part of your sexual personality that you don't like. If you have an explicit dream of suicide, don't worry that you're about to take your own life. You are expressing your unconscious dissatisfaction with some aspect of your sexual behavior, and you are trying to stamp it out. How you interpret your killing dream may depend on what method you employ to commit your murder. If you shoot your lover with a gun, you are trying to close your relationship without risking any further involvement. If you stab him with a knife or dagger (or scissors), you are making a last effort to show your lover that there may still be some hope for you. Sexually, at least, if not in any other way.

King

When you have a sexual dream in which a king appears, he may represent your father, or some other man you respect and admire. All dreams of kings and queens, whether they're erotic or not, show a desire to have establishment approval and recognition, and illicit lovers sometimes dream that they're meeting kings and queens at court to receive royal confirmation of their love affair. Princes and lesser male royalty may represent men whom you find attractive, but whose personalities have not made sufficient impact on you for you to consider them seriously as lovers.

Kiss

As in waking life, kisses in erotic dreams have various different meanings. But unlike waking kisses, dream kisses are complicated messages of love and sexuality, and can tell you quite subtle things about the person you're kissing and yourself. If you kiss a man long and deep, and you push your tongue into his mouth, you are prepared to commit yourself to him sexually, but you want him to do the same to you. If you kiss a man on the cheek, you're demonstrating your friendship but not your love. If you kiss a man on his penis, but don't let it lead to fellatio, you're showing that you find him sexually attractive, and you respect his sexuality, but you're not prepared to commit yourself to an intimate relationship. If you kiss a man's bottom or anus, then beware of your feelings for him. The dream means exactly what it seems — you're kissing his ass. Dreams of foot-kissing have similar interpretations. If you have a sexual dream in which you kiss your lover and leave marks or stigmata on his skin, then you may be feeling too possessive about him, and you want to show everyone that he's yours.

Knight

If you have a sexual dream in which a knight in armor appears, you may be having romantic visions of what an ideal sexual relationship could be like. If the armor is white and shining, you are entranced by the idea of a man coming into your life and sweeping you off your feet. If it's black, you find men sexually attractive but you are frightened of becoming involved with them. If it's rusty, you may be dreaming that your one-time ideal man has let you down, and that your relationship with him is gradually showing signs of wear. If you dream that you have a sexual affair with a knight in armor, only to discover that his suit of armor is empty, you are probably beginning to find your present sexual relationship is little more than a hollow sham.

Knot

Knots appear in all kinds of dreams as visual manifestations of your sexual problems. But they have other meanings as well. If you and your lover are tied together ('a lovers' knot'), it can mean that you feel closely bound to him, either willingly or unwillingly. If your lover ties you up, you may have a latent masochistic streak in you, and you're looking for the kind of relationship in which your own desires are dominated by his. If you tie him up, then you're probably dreaming that you're easily able to control your lover's desires, and that you have a mildly sadistic vein in your sexual personality. You're the sort of girl who constantly challenges a man's masculinity and derives malicious pleasure from confusing him and 'tying him up in knots'.

L

Labia

Your vaginal labia (the lips that guard your hole against dust, dirt and inquisitive wasps) can sometimes appear in your sexual dreams in different guises. This is not usually because you're embarrassed or shy about them, but because they are not a prominent and visible part of your body, and your mental conception of what they look like is often different from what they actually do look like. Unlike many primitive societies, the female sexual organs are no longer displayed openly and provocatively (except in overtight ski pants as worn by some of the more generously proportioned matrons of the Midwest). That means you are not familiar with the way you and other women look close up. Labia can appear in your sexual dreams as flowers, as the flaps of envelopes, as ordinary lips, as purse clasps, or even (as in one girl's dream) as the complete neck of a hot water bag. Women have fewer erotic dreams about labia than men, for obvious reasons. But just as it's possible to judge a man's attitude towards your vagina by checking what dream image he has of your labia (is he afraid of it, and sees it as a snarling mouth?), you can evaluate your own attitude to your sexual organs by seeing what you think of them. If your labia appears as petals and other soft and attractive things, you are probably proud of and content with your sexuality. If they appear as awkward, ugly or incongruous, then you may have some doubts and fears about your physical self.

Lesbians

Author Jodi Lawrence once suggested that 'in increasing numbers, young feminists are turning to homosexuality for their sexual release, and many state this sexual choice is due to their distaste for the stereotyped implications of man-woman relationships.' When you have an erotic dream in which you have a lesbian affair, it's possible that you're doing just this – escaping the pressures and frustrations of heterosexual love by turning to someone who will understand your problems and not impose any unwelcome sexual roles on you. It's a fantasy, of course, because everybody imposes unwelcome sexual roles on everybody else, and most successful sexual relationships are only a working compromise between two individual concepts of ecstasy. But a lesbian dream may show that you want a rest from the strains of man-woman sex without resorting to total celibacy. It may also show that you have some lesbian tendencies (probably under strict control during your waking life), or that you have narcissistic feelings about your own eroticism. This is a curious lesbian dream from a 22-year-old Detroit hostess, which combines both self-love and homosexual love:

I'm alone in a dark room, and I'm sitting astride an upright chair in front of an oval mirror. My hair is about the only thing that shines in the whole room. It's very gloomy. One of those days when you think that perhaps the world is going to end. I'm wearing a black wasp-waisted corselette, and lace-up boots like you see those women wearing in cowboy movies. 'Hi there, Miss Stacey, this is a fine whorehouse you got yourself here.' – that kind of thing. I look at my face in the mirror and although the girl in the mirror must be me, she has different color eyes – brown – and her hair is mid-blond, while mine is more coppery. I look closer. She's wearing a corselette, too, but hers is dark brown, like a Bunny costume. My cunt is showing, and I look in the mirror at this other girl's cunt, to see what color her cunt hair is, and it's blonde, while mine is really dark. I get frightened. But it seems like a sexy situation, too. I walk up to the mirror and the girl walks up towards me, just like a mirror image would. I kiss her, very carefully. I can feel her lips and taste her lipstick. I put my arms around her and I can feel her breasts pressing against my breasts, and her pubic hair touching mine, and her thighs against my thighs. We kiss again, and this time we run our tongues across each other's lips. I run my hand down her back and feel her naked ass. It's warm and firm. I can hardly believe it. I slide my fingers very gently into her cunt, and it feels just like a real cunt, so it must be real. I say: 'I love you ... you're some other girl.' And she's just about to say something back to me when I wake up. I'm all wound up in my sheets, I'm baking hot, and my fingers are halfway up my cunt.

If you have an unpleasant sexual dream in which you are assaulted by a lesbian, or in which you take part in a lesbian activity which you don't enjoy, then your dreaming mind is making an effort to repress your lesbian tendencies. If you try not to feel worried or guilty about any marginal homosexual feelings that you might have, then you probably won't have any more nasty dreams about them. As I've said before, we all have some traces of homosexuality in us, and unless you're having an out-and-out mental struggle about your sexual leanings, there is nothing to worry about. If you have a dream in which you discover that a girl friend of yours is a lesbian, your mind may be pointing out things about her which you had never consciously noticed. But don't judge her on the strength of your dream alone. If it really makes a difference to you if she's lesbian or not, make your mind up from what you see of her in waking life.

Letter

According to ancient dream divinations, an unopened letter represents virginity, and the act of opening that letter represents defloration. The appearance of a letter in your sexual dream may also mean that you are being reminded of some information that your unconscious mind has taken in, and which you have so far chosen to ignore. If you refuse to read a letter in your dream, you are deliberately turning a blind eye to some sexual problem.

Lion

If you have an erotic dream in which a lion appears – or in which you are having sex with a lion – you may be dreaming about a strong and passionate man in your life. Ancient dream books all agree that the lion is a symbol of whirlwind sexual success, of power and strength. If you dream you are attacked by a lion, you are dreaming that some wilful man is sweeping you off your feet and into bed. But if he bites and mauls you, his passion might be causing chaos in your life, with disastrous results for your sexual equilibrium and peace of mind.

Liquids

Freud believed that our sleeping minds sometimes substitute inoffensive liquids such as milk or wine for sexual fluids. I have come across several dreams in which erotic liquids take on some peculiar forms, and it may be possible to interpret your attitude towards your current sexual involvement by determining what you feel about the sexual liquids in your dream. A 25-year-old Nebraska girl wrote and told me that she had dreams in which she swallowed her husband's semen and it 'tasted like nectar.' She was obviously content with her relationship and with oral sex. But a New York advertising artist told me that whenever she dreamed about fellatio, her lover's penis looked and tasted like a Hungarian salami, and his come emerged like 'thin, garlicky blood.' Not very nice, really. Some women have an uncertain relationship with their own bodily fluids, and are embarrassed by excessive vaginal lubrication, discharges and menstrual blood. In sexual dreams, this uncertainty can sometimes be translated into out-and-out revulsion, and I have read dream reports in which women have variously imagined that their vaginas were discharging molasses, minestrone soup stinking of Parmesan cheese, mud, olive oil, and Irish stew. If you have sexual dreams in which you imagine you have peculiar vaginal discharges, try to examine your attitudes towards the physical side of your femininity, and see if you can't perhaps come to more comfortable terms with it.

M

Magic

Because they don't have to obey the laws of gravity or logic, dreams are crowded with apparently magical events.

But in some erotic dreams, you may find that you or your lover are actually able to work magic, and this has a meaning all of its own. It usually indicates that you are vexed by sexual difficulties, and you're looking for a quick and easy way out of them. Here's the 'magic' dream of a 41-year-old married woman from Long Island:

I seem to have fetched the groceries from the store down the street. My husband Stan is lying on the bed, and he calls through the bedroom door: 'Come to bed, June, I want you.' I walk into the bedroom and he's holding his penis in his hand. It's standing up, and it looks so big it's almost like a great red tree. Well, I know in my dream that Stan has problems getting erections, so I quickly take off my clothes and go toward the bed. Just when I'm trying to get his penis inside me, though, it sinks down and goes small again. I feel that same disappointment like I do in real life. But this time, in the dream, I don't seem worried. I go back to my grocery sack, and I take out a jar of dried herbs, and I bring them back to the bedroom. I sprinkle some on the top of Stan's penis, and I kind of make circles in the air with my hands, and his penis starts to rise up, like it's magic. Stan's pleased, and I'm pleased. We start to make love, and it actually works. It's beautiful. We both reach a climax, and we lie back there all satisfied, and I know that whenever I want Stan to have himself an erection, all I have to do is use the herbs and the magic gestures.

This dream is more than a little poignant. For more than five years, this woman had been unable to have satisfactory intercourse because of her husband's unrelenting impotence, and there's no doubt that this was a 'wishful thinking' dream. On the whole, the sexual magic you perform in your erotic dreams seems to be an expression of those far-fetched desires which you know, in waking life, could never come true. 'I wish my husband's penis would stay hard forever . . .' 'I wish I could have enormous breasts . . .' 'I wish I could see through men's clothes . . .'

Masturbation

Your dreams of masturbation will vary according to your attitudes toward self-stimulation. If you feel guilty about masturbation, or offended by it, then your dreams will be full of furtive and embarrassing sexual moments. You will have dreams of being caught masturbating by other people, of being ridiculed because of your masturbation, and of conflicts and arguments about masturbation. But if you enjoy masturbation, and it does not disturb you or make you feel ashamed, you will have dreams of using masturbation to fulfill yourself, of openly masturbating to the applause of other people, and of masturbating in front of your lover. So many women masturbate in so many different ways that it's impossible to touch on anything more than a fraction of masturbation dreams. There are three principal methods of female masturbation – stimulating the clitoris with the fingers or a vibrator, squeezing the thighs together and arousing the whole genital area, and inserting fingers or other objects into the vagina in a simulation of intercourse. If you have sexy dreams of activities which resemble your personal method of masturbation, then you are probably dreaming about masturbation proper. We mentioned earlier that an activity like sewing can be a dream substitute for diddling yourself. Here's another 'substitute' dream from an 18-year-old girl from Newark, New Jersey:

I dreamed that I was sitting in class, in college, and I suddenly thought to myself, 'I have a terrible urge to make cookies.' I left the class and went down to the cookery class. They didn't seem to mind that I walked from one class to another. The cookery teacher was talking to some of the other girls there, so I went over and started to make the mixture for the cookies. I knew I had to roll the cookies out, so I sat on a stool, and I pulled my skirt up, right up to my panties, and I laid pieces of cookie mix all along the insides of my thighs. Then I put a rolling pin upright between my legs and pressed my legs together so that the rolling pin traveled from my knees to my thighs, rolling out the pastry as it went. I pressed my legs together faster and faster, and the rolling pin kept touching up against my panties, and giving me a strange tingle between the legs. I didn't seem to worry that anybody was watching me doing this, because as far as I was concerned I was making cookies and that was all.

If you have constant dreams of masturbation, even when you're married or involved in a long-term affair, then you may feel that you're not sexually satisfied, and that you need to seek fulfillment elsewhere. They may mean, too, that you feel sexually isolated from the men in your life, and that somehow they're failing to involve you emotionally in your joint relationship. If you masturbate in your dreams in front of other people, you may feel that your sexual opinions and attitudes shock other people, or at least disturb them, but you derive personal pleasure out of your sexual behavior, and you don't really care what other people think. If you dream that you're masturbating in front of your husband or lover, you may feel that he doesn't understand your sexual needs clearly enough, and that he needs to be shown what will turn you on. You may also be showing him that you're sexually independent, and that you feel he's trying to become too dominant in your sexual relationship. When you have dreams about masturbating with unusual or painful objects, you're possibly showing that you have fears about your sexual desires, or that you're anxious about the size and appearance of your lover's penis, or that you're deliberately hurting yourself as a penance for having lustful thoughts and feelings. It depends what the object is. One Santa Barbara woman said she dreamed she was masturbating herself with a long-handled jeweled comb, and that it was 'delicious agony.' She didn't consciously remember the comb, but when she mentioned it to her widowed father, he reminded her that it used to belong to her late mother, who had always been stern and disapproving on sexual and moral subjects. Probably the oddest masturbation-object dream I have come across came from a 27-year-old New York woman who dreamed she was masturbating with paperback books by riffling the pages against her clitoris. Don't get any ideas about this book.

Matches

To have a dream in which you are striking matches is probably a dream of regular, enjoyable intercourse. The matches themselves can represent the penis, according to some dream diviners – although I personally think they lack the proportions and meatiness of full-fledged phallic symbols. Lighting matches may also represent provocative sexual behavior and flirtations.

Moon

The moon, when it rises in your sexual dreams, is a very powerful symbol of dominant femininity. It can represent your mother, and her influence on you, but more often it stands for the female strength that is within you, and the sisterhood of women to which you belong. In moonlight, a woman is in her natural feminine element ('moonlight becomes you,' as the song says) and to dream of sex under the waxing moon is to dream that your sexual personality is very strong, and your sexual relationship is running completely in your favor. If the moon is sinking or waning, then your sex life may be fading. A thumbnail moon is sometimes interpreted as a sign of optimism and hope for women who are seeking a new lover.

Mountains

If mountains appear in your erotic dreams, they may represent sexual obstacles and problems which you fear may be insurmountable. But, as we have seen from actual dreams, they may also represent your own body or the body of your lover. Try and recall the topography of the mountains, to see if it resembles any possible part of the human body. In one cute sexual dream, a 16-year-old-girl thought that her boyfriend's face (acne and all) was carved on Mount Rushmore along with the presidents, and she spent half the dream searching for the place where his penis was carved, so that they could make love.

Music

It is fascinating how often music features in sexual dreams – tunes that can actually be named and remembered. Sometimes the title or the theme of the tune is relevant to what is happening in the dream itself. Sometimes it's just a piece of music that the dreamer has got stuck in her mind. Music may often represent the pattern of your sexual relationship, and you should try to 'listen' closely to detect if the music is harmonious or discordant. Since music is capable of conveying very subtle shades of emotion, you may learn a great deal from the music in your dream. Happy music reflects a happy relationship; trite music reflects a shallow relationship; sad music reflects a dolorous relationship.

N

Needles

To have a sexual dream in which you are pricked by a needle suggests that you might have recently had an awkward or irritating sexual experience. But if you have stored the needle away in your lapel, or in a piece of fabric, you feel you have your lover's sexual desires well under control.

Nipples

Nipples sometimes take on curious forms and meanings in sexual dreams. If you dream that your nipples have eyes, you may have unconscious fears that someone is taking sexual advantage of you, and that your body is keeping its own watch on what's going on. If you dream that your nipples are buttons or switches, you are simply dreaming that you can be aroused by a man touching your nipples – 'turning you on'. If you have dreams in which your nipples are painted or decorated, you are probably trying to draw attention to your breasts for some reason, but you may also be trying to draw attention away from your face or another part of your body. Dreams of decorating your nipples with lipstick or paint are indications of a sensual personality, and also a personality that is quite orally oriented. If you dream that you have no nipples at all, you may be anxious about your sexual ability and attractiveness, and also confused about the way in which your sexual relationship is developing. One New York woman, an aggressive sexual personality, dreamed that her nipples were the muzzles of guns, and that she could fire at men she found desirable to seduce and conquer them.

Noise

If there is a distinctive or irritating noise in the background of your sexual dream, then something may be worrying you that you don't consciously want to face up to. Try and isolate the noise, and decide if it corresponds to any of your sexual problems. Police and fire sirens may be warning you of trouble in your relationship; irregular motor noises (see *engine*) may be pointing out some defect in the harmony of your sexual activities. Be sensible about the interpretation of noises, though. Usually, it's only the noticeable and unusual noise that has any symbolic meaning. And remember that, during your dreams, noises can filter into your mind from the street outside, or your lover snoring next to you, or a rattling radiator.

Nose

In erotic dreams, noses can sometimes represent the male penis, and if you dream about a man with a prominent nose, you may be thinking about sexual intercourse with him. This interpretation is particularly likely if you dream that the nose is growing, or that it's ejaculating fluid. Noses can also represent intuition, and the feeling that there's something amiss in your sexual relationship, especially if they're sniffing.

Nudity

You will frequently find that you're naked in your sexual dreams, but *how* and *why* and *where* you're naked are the all-important factors in making a clear interpretation. If you dream that you're naked in bed with your lover, then your nudity is perfectly normal and natural. You wouldn't expect to make love to him with your clothes on, and if you did, your dream might be telling you something important about your relationship, like 'Am I secretly embarrassed about sharing my body with him?' If you have dreams in which you appear nude in public, the meaning of your dream will depend on how you feel about it. If you're ashamed and embarrassed, your unconscious mind is revealing your guilt about your current sexual behavior. If you're carefree and merry about it, then you're confident about your sexual relationships to the point of exhibitionism. If you have dreams in which you appear naked at formal parties and functions, you may be trying to convince the establishment that your sexual conduct is acceptable and even praiseworthy, or you may be cocking a snook at their stuffiness and prudery. It depends on what you do in your dream. If you feel anxious about your nudity, and you want to hide, then you are showing how little erotic bravado you have, and you're probably the kind of girl who shies away from blatant sexual approaches from men. If you have persistent sexual dreams in which you show yourself off in front of other people, there may be a sexy streak in you that's trying to find some way out – so try dressing sexily in real life, and see if the real you is more daring than ever imagined. If you have persistent dreams in which you're embarrassed about your nudity, then there's obviously something wrong in your sex life, and it would be worth your while to find out what it is. Here's an interesting excerpt from a nudity dream in which a 32-year-old Houston, Texas, woman is showing that she desires to be desired, but is still afraid to take the plunge and act provocatively herself:

I was walking along the street, and there were different sculptures and statues standing around. One of the statues was a nude statue of me. I knew it was me, and I stood close by, watching how other people reacted to it. Several men came up and caressed the statue's breasts, and some of them said what a

–

sexy statue it was. I felt quite an urge to go up and say: 'That's me, that statue – that's based exactly on me,' but I didn't have the nerve. Then I thought if maybe I took off my clothes, and stood quite still, then men would come and caress me, just like they did to my statue. I was about to do that when I woke up.

If you dream that other people are naked in normal surroundings – your next-door neighbor, for instance, or your boss at work – then you are showing a natural curiosity in their maleness. It means that you've noticed them as sexual people, even though you may never have consciously considered an affair with them, or never would.

Numbers

According to some dream divinations, numbers have a sexual significance. The number 1 is symbolic of the male penis, and the number 0 stands for the female vagina. The number 10 therefore represents man and woman together. The number 8 may symbolize breasts, or an endless situation out of which there seems to be no escape. The numbers 6 and 9, apart from their obvious sexual significance in the oral act of sixty-nine, stand for sexual and emotional upheaval. Numbers in dreams tend to be very elusive: I had a sexual dream myself in which, everytime I dialed a digit on the telephone, the entire arrangement of numbers on the dial was changed around. But try and recall your dream numbers – they may have a significance that will only become apparent when you dream about them again.

Nuts

If you have a sexual dream in which nuts appear, then you're probably dreaming about male testicles and particularly about the sperm they create. It may be that you're beginning to feel like having a child.

Nymphomania

As I pointed out in *1,001 Erotic Dreams Interpreted*: 'Dreams that appear to be dreams of nymphomaniac behavior are often only excessive in comparison to the limited amount of sex that our civilized way of life allows us to have during the day. As Masters and Johnson have shown, women are frequently capable of having orgasm after orgasm until they collapse from sheer exhaustion, and to have sex as often as your body permits can hardly be considered to be overdoing things. There is far more social and personal distress caused in the United States by overeating than by overscrewing.' If you have what appears to be an incredible number of sexual acts in your dreams, your unconscious mind is simply revealing how much sex you could have (mentally rather than physically) if you didn't have any restrictions on your sexual activity at all. If you have a dream in which people disapprove of your numerous sexual acts, however, you are probably feeling guilty about your present sexual activities, and you have a suppressed notion that you're acting like a whore. Try and root that notion out, because it may have an adverse effect on your relationship. If, like true nymphomaniacs, you have a great deal of sex but can never quite manage to reach an orgasm, you are probably dreaming that your sex life is unfulfilling. Not necessarily physically, but in some way that your waking mind won't admit to. You may also be dreaming that, even though you're attracted to the man in your life, you're not prepared to commit yourself to him totally. You may be nervous or worried about your sexual technique, or you may be afraid of becoming pregnant. Sometimes, women dream about uncontrollable nymphomaniac behavior because they want to lay the responsibility for their own strong sexual desires on to a clinical condition. 'I couldn't help myself, doctor. I just had to have it.' Here's a nymphomaniac dream from a 24-year-old Detroit girl whose prudish husband had made her feel that her sexual appetite was in some way abnormal:

Henry's at work, so I sneak out of the back of the house and start up the Pinto. I drive out to a big factory that I've noticed on the edge of town. I drive through the gates and I park the car and get out. The factory door is open, and I walk in without anyone asking me what I'm doing. It's an auto plant, and there are men working all around on the assembly line. The noise is tremendous, but I don't mind it. I know just what I've come for. I walk into the middle of the shop floor, and I take down my jeans and my panties. All I'm wearing is a small studded denim jacket and shoes. The men stop work and they crowd around. They're beautiful men. Real American car-worker types. They're big and they're strong and they're greasy. I lie down on a pile of sacks and tools, and the men come up to me with their pricks all ready. I close my eyes. I know that I'm asleep, and that I'm soon going to wake up, but I can still lie back there and enjoy the feeling of being taken by so many men. I cling on to the sacks and I cling on to the dream. I'm half-awake, half in the dream and half in my own bed. I must have had about five or six men, and when they faded away altogether, my thighs were covered in engine grease and the sperm was pouring out of me like a knocked-over carton of cream.

O

Odor

Dreams can make use of all five senses, and you can 'smell' perfumes and food and flowers in your dreams as distinctly as you can 'hear' or 'feel' or 'see'. A lurking perfume can often tell you something about your sexual dream that is not at first apparent. If you're making love to your husband or steady lover, are you sure that he smells like the man he should be? Or is he wearing the aftershave that you always associated with another man in your life? Sometimes a dream smell will be making a comment or a joke about the main action of the dream. A Los Angeles woman dreamed that she was talking to her lover, and that he was asking her to marry him, but all the time she could distinctly detect the lingering odor of fish. Her dreaming mind was simply saying that whatever her lover had in mind 'smelt fishy'. In erotic dreams, sexual odors frequently smell different from the way they do in real life. This may be because we have all been conditioned to respond to artificial fragrances rather than the natural smells of the human body. See if you can identify the odors that arouse you in dreams, because they could tell you something about your sexual personality. Do you prefer fresh, lemony smells, or heavy, Eastern fragrances? Are you sexually brisk and active, or are you sensual and languid?

Oil

If you have a sexual dream of oil, you are usually dreaming of semen or sexual lubricants, but the lubricants may have a deeper significance than just aids to successful intercourse. They may represent the understanding and agreement that allows your whole affair to run smoothly.

Onions

Onions have extraordinary properties as vegetables, and they also have extraordinary meanings in dreams. If you have a sexual dream in which you are peeling onions, and shedding tears because of it, it can mean that you are breaking up your present sexual relationship, but only pretending to feel upset about it. Onions were generally thought to be a good omen by ye olde dream diviners. They may also appear as breasts or testicles, but because of their obviously layered form, they are more often associated with complex sexual relationships in which one layer of emotion hides another and yet another.

Organ

Dreams of organs playing are interpreted by ancient dream books as standing for continuing sexual satisfaction. Enough jokes are made about organs for them to appear in your dreams as visual puns for penises, but you must also remember that organ music is commonly associated with weddings, prayers and other ceremonial occasions.

Orgy

Erotic dreams of orgies are comparatively unusual, especially among women, and when you do have one it usually has a serious and significant meaning. If you have an orgy dream in which you are involved in a sexual menage with your husband or lover, then you may be trying to show them that you have erotic needs which they haven't yet been able to satisfy. You are demonstrating that you are capable of having sex with them, and more besides. Many women dream that they are having sex with several men, but on closer examination, they realize that every man in the dream was a different manifestation of their own husband. This indicates that they are bored with their sex lives, but they are not yet prepared to seek their sexual fulfillment elsewhere. If you have a dream in which you are involved in an orgy with total strangers, then you are probably feeling deep dissatisfaction with your present sexual relationship, and you are thinking about going out into the sexual marketplace again and looking for new men. Orgy dreams in which you are the undisputed center of attention may show that you crave more sexual interest and excitement from your lover. Here's an orgy dream which expressed just that for a 29-year-old East Hampton girl:

I was on a bus. I don't know where we were all going. There was me and a whole company of men with black, center-parted hair and black tuxedos. We could've been in Oklahoma or someplace like that. It looked like the boondocks, wherever it was. There were some other girls there, and they were wearing Twenties clothes, with long strings of beads, and they were dancing up and down the aisle of the bus. When they kicked their legs high, I could see their cunts. They weren't wearing any panties. Then I looked down at all the men, and their pricks were lying on their laps like German sausages. The girls and the men all began to climb up into the baggage racks along the side of the bus, and they were actually fucking. I could see them. I could see pricks going into cunts, and I could even hear them, panting and gasping and squealing. Then two of the men took hold of me, and I went all exotic and sexy, licking my lips and pouting and sticking my bust out. They pulled off my clothes, and I posed and put my hands on my hips like Marlene Dietrich and really showed myself off. The men raised me over their heads, and carried me down the whole length of the bus, and everybody in the whole bus had to stick their fingers into my cunt, and then take them out and lick them. After that, I did an exotic dance down the bus, and the men all waved their pricks at me, and the girls all swung their pearls. I heard a bell ringing, and someone was saying *Tuxedo Lake, Tuxedo Lake*, and I was just about to say, *well, we can't be here already*, and I woke up.

Oven

If you have sexual dreams in which you are baking, or putting cakes or food into the oven, then you may have suspicions that your lovemaking has made you pregnant.

They may simply mean that you have a suppressed desire to have children, but the general atmosphere of the dream will make this clear. One women told me that she had a dream in which she placed a large pan of bread dough into the oven, and then very deliberately turned the temperature dial to nine. I don't see how any dream could get more representative of pregnancy than that.

P

Paralysis

If you have a sexual dream in which you imagine you are paralyzed, or rooted to the spot, then there is something in your sexual life which both attracts and disgusts you. It may be a sexual act that your lover has suggested. It may be your lover himself. Whatever it is, you may not be able to rid yourself of your dreams until you decide what you are going to do about it.

Pearls

When pearls appear in sexual dreams, they may represent drops of semen, or they may represent material wealth. If you dream that you are having sex wearing a pearl necklace, it may be that you think you are lowering yourself by having intercourse with whoever is making love to you in your dream. A dream of breaking a pearl necklace can sometimes represent a sexual climax, although for some reason there is a sense of loss connected with it. Are you afraid that by surrendering yourself sexually to the man in your life, you might have given up some of your independence and freedom?

Penis

When a penis appears in a sexual dream, it's usually fairly obvious that it's a penis, no matter how it's dressed up or disguised. The interesting question is *why* you see a penis as an umbrella or a carrot or a loaf of bread, or in whatever strange form you imagine it. If you have a dream in which you see penises that are very heavily disguised as other things, then it's possible that the male sexual organs embarrass or worry you. Don't try to see penises in everything that's rounded and pointed – you'll know what's a penis and what isn't by the way you feel about it in your dream. An elderly woman I spoke to said that she dreamed she was back in Cyprus, and was hurrying past a minaret because it made her feel uncomfortable and odd. If you have a dream in which you see a penis as something prickly and awkward, then you may have hidden fears that sex or sexual relationships will be just the same way. If you dream that a penis is too big and hard for you, you may either be worried that your lover is going to be too difficult for you to handle, or you may be the kind of girl who likes to be dominated and hurt by her sexual partners. If you dream that a penis is too short or too thin, you may be concerned that your lover isn't going to satisfy you enough. If the penis is very noticeable (a strange color, perhaps, or an odd shape), then you may be alarmed about your lover trying unusual and deviant sex techniques on you. Sometimes, the penis you see in your dreams will have a life of its own – its own mouth and its own eyes. Dreams like this sometimes indicate that you are attracted to your lover but dissatisfied or anxious about his sexual response. You see his penis as an independent being who doesn't like you, even though your lover does. Be warned that the behavior of a penis exactly reflects the desires of its owner. If you acquire a penis yourself in your dreams, it is usually a sign that you feel the need to dominate your sexual partner and direct the course of your sexual relationship yourself. Sometimes a penis will behave in remarkable ways in your dreams, and this behavior is usually a clear indication of how you feel about sex with your husband or lover. Here's a penis dream from a 30-year-old wife from San Diego, California:

I dreamed I was washing my car when my next-door neighbor, Mr Ronson, came up and started speaking to me. I was wearing short shorts, and they were soaked in water from the hose, and I was a little worried that Mr Ronson would be able to see right through them, and see my pubic hair. All of a sudden, I felt something warm touching my bottom. I turned around, and Mr Ronson's penis had sprung out of his pants, and grown about a foot and was touching me on the bottom. I tried to be nice, and tell him that I ought to get on with washing the car, but instead of picking up the hose, I picked up this long warm penis of his, and it went extremely stiff – so stiff that I could hardly manage to point it at my car. I rubbed it up and down, and it poured sperm all over the windshield of my car. There must've been two gallons of it. Then I was worried that my husband would come home, and find out I'd been unfaithful. The sperm was like rubber solution, and I couldn't get it off the glass for love nor money. Mr Ronson ran off down the street, holding his balls in one hand and his penis in the other, which had gone down to the right size by then. It was a very silly dream, but it embarrassed me, and I've never told my husband about it.

Perversions

During a sexual dream, it's often difficult to decide what's perversion and what isn't, since so many of the sexual events that take place have unusual or fetishistic associations. One girl dreamed that she was pushing cold cooked squash into her vagina and wooden spoons up her anus, and she was terrified that someone was going to find out. Another woman told me she had a dream in which she was addicted to cold cream, and spent hours smothering her naked body and her hair with it. Unless you have an overwhelming urge to play out these erotic perversions for real, you have nothing to worry about. These dreams are simply expressions of remote anxieties about sex and sexual behavior, and don't mean for one moment that you have any genuine aberration.

Pockets

In erotic dreams, pockets may often represent female sexual organs. If there is something concealed inside the pocket, then it's possible that you have a sexual secret which you've been hiding from your lover and even from yourself. A young New York secretary dreamed that her boss was trying to push his penis into her pocket, but when he did so, it was painfully cut by pieces of smashed glass. She admitted that she had been flirting with her boss, but that she was about to become engaged to another man (the smashed glass was broken windshield glass that she had seen in the road recently — it had reminded her of engagement diamonds).

Polygamy

When you dream of living with more than one husband, you are probably showing that you are tired of your present partner, but that you are conventional enough to want your sexual variations within the bounds of marriage. Such a dream indicates that you are highly sexed, but not promiscuous, and that you are the kind of woman who will go a long way to appear respectable.

Prostitute

If you have a sexual dream in which you are a prostitute — offering sex of any kind in return for reward of any kind —

then you may be unsure of your sexual attractiveness, and you are trying to make certain that men find you sexy by demanding visible proof of their feelings. The dream may also indicate that you are disillusioned with the romantic side of your sexual relationship, and you feel that your sex life has become an unglamorous trading arrangement – intercourse in return for security and housekeeping money.

Puzzles

When you have sexual dreams in which you are obliged to solve puzzles, you may be suffering from serious sexual difficulties in your marriage or affair that have to be sorted out before you can continue your relationship with happiness and equilibrium. Dream puzzles may be as simple as those plastic toys where you have to roll a ball-bearing into a small hole, or they may be elaborate and complicated beyond reasonable understanding. One woman's sexual difficulties were very candidly outlined in this erotic dream puzzle, which she dreamed about night after night for weeks on end.

My husband, Lloyd, and I were both sitting in the bedroom. We were both naked, and I had the feeling that there were 'no illusions between us.' I guess we had been married long enough not to have any fanciful ideas about what we were or what we might have been. We were cross-legged on the rug, and between us there was a puzzle made out of wires and crystals. The idea of the puzzle seemed to be that you had to stare at a small crystal until the vibrations from your mind heated it up to the point where it glowed. Then, while it was still glowing, you had to mentally direct it up and around this wire structure, which was very complex and full of traps and diversions. I knew that it was vitally important for me to do this puzzle right, because the rules seemed to be that we couldn't have sexual intercourse until the puzzle was solved. The trouble was, every time I stared at the crystal I began to get turned on, and when I was turned on I put my hand down between my legs and started to masturbate. As soon as I masturbated, I lost my concentration and the crystal went dim again. I think now that it was a dream about the whole way that our marriage was going. We lived from day to day. If we'd tried to get our minds together and sort out what was really amiss with us, we maybe would've gotten someplace. But we lived for our own self-gratification, and once we were gratified, we lost our will to do anything at all.

Q

Queen

Erotic dreams which include a queen figure may indicate that you feel sexually dominated or overshadowed by your mother. Queens can also symbolize strong sexual rivals or the wife of your lover if he's married to someone else.

Questions

If your sexual dreams are full of questions, you're obviously feeling uncertain about your present relationship. You will often learn more by looking at the questions themselves than by trying to supply answers to them. The very fact that you're asking: 'How much do I love my husband?' suggests that there's some doubt that you love him at all. If the question is incomprehensible, or seems to bear no relation to anything within the dream at all, it's sometimes possible to interpret the entire dream as a question. 'Here is a situation,' your mind is saying, 'now, what do you think about it?'

Quilt

If you have a sexual dream in which you are making love on a patchwork quilt, then you may feel that your erotic relationship has become domesticated and boring, and lacks sophistication. On the other hand, you may feel that you want all those qualities that patchwork quilts represent – coziness and home craftsmanship – and in that case a quilt dream is a dream of 'wishful thinking'. On the whole, though, patchwork quilts seem to appear mostly in dreams of sexual uncertainty, impatience and confusion.

R

Rain

When rain falls in erotic dreams, it can sometimes suggest urine or semen. But it can also represent hopes of a new start in your sexual relationship, and the gradual refreshment of your sexual ideals.

Rape

For a detailed discussion of rape dreams, consult the chapter on ten common erotic dreams. But remember that suggestions of rape can appear in your dreams without anyone actually having forcible sex with you. If the idea of being raped has a marginal fascination for you, look out for symbols in your dreams like rusty keys being forced into locks, pestles being mashed into mortars, dough being kneaded by brawny fists, and boots being plunged into mud. A rape dream can even take the form of strange and terrifying men trying to break into your home, or any kind of intrusion into your personal privacy.

Razor

When razors appear in erotic dreams, they usually seem to represent some kind of difficult decision that you have to make in your sexual life. If you have a dream in which your husband or lover is shaving, you may be questioning his virility, or you may be feeling that he is turning over a new leaf and changing his ideas about you.

Riding

Horseback riding has always had erotic connotations, and when you have dreams in which you are deriving sexual pleasure from riding, it can show that you delight in being dominating and forceful in your present sexual relationship. Your dream may be even more explicit – you may actually be riding on your lover's back. This is a sexual proclivity which, when it occurs in real life, is known as *equus eroticus* – literally, the sexy horse. Your sense of sexual superiority will be shown in your dream by the way you ride your 'horse', how hard you whip and spur him, and whether you're prepared to reward him at the end of your ride.

I was walking a huge gray horse over the open prairie. There was no one else around, and I was riding the horse bareback. At first I was dressed in stetson and jeans and a checkered shirt, but as the dream continued I lost all my clothes and ended up nude. I looked at my watch and realized 'there isn't much tick left in the old thing.' I coaxed the horse into trotting, and I was moving up and down on its back with a slow and easy motion. The feeling excited me, and I clicked my tongue to make the horse go faster. When he cantered faster, he excited me even more, and I was sweating all over my naked body and screaming at the horse to hurry. We galloped miles and miles across this wide-open prairie, and soon the horse was going so fast that I couldn't stand the tension that was building up in me. It was just like a massive orgasm – the kind of orgasm that hits you like a log on the back of your neck and makes you feel you've been killed. I could feel this orgasm winding up and winding up, tighter and tighter, and I was gritting my teeth. The horse was even making my breasts jiggle up and down, which gave me even more of a sexual sensation. That horse went like a machine, up-down, up-down, up-down, up-down. I dug my nails in its neck and shrieked. I made it go even faster, so that finally my orgasm rose up and tore me to pieces. I woke up because my father came into the room to ask if I was all right, I'd been making such a noise in my sleep.

That was the riding dream of a 17-year-old girl from Dallas, Texas. She was an attractive girl, with a great many boyfriends, and she admitted that she tended to treat her steadies 'like a stable of stallions.' See also *horse*.

River

If there is a river in the background of your sexual dream, it may symbolize the progress of your sexual relationship. If it's wide, lazy and slow-moving, then your relationship will be developing slowly and surely. But if it's fast-running and full of rocks, then you can expect your relationship to shape up the same way. To dream that you're swimming or washing yourself in a river is an indication that you want to make a fresh start.

Road

A road, like a river, may represent the progress of your latest affair. But – unlike rivers – roads arrive in towns and specific places. If you have a sexual dream in which you are traveling and never reach your destination, you may be feeling sexually unfulfilled. If you do arrive, but feel disappointed at your destination, then you may be getting regular sexual attention, but it may be too unimaginative or routine for you. If you arrive someplace exciting and glamorous, then your sexual relationship is going well. 'I used to have dreams about traveling from town to town when I was first married,' said a 34-year-old New Hampshire woman. 'The towns were always the same.

Full of suburban houses, small gardens, dull municipal halls. Then I divorced and married my second husband, and the dreams changed altogether. I found myself in fantastic cities, almost like Oz or something, and I began to understand just what my first marriage had lacked.'

Running

If you have erotic dreams in which you are running for the sake of running, then you may be dreaming about masturbation. If you are running away from a man, then you are possibly trying to evade the responsibilities of a sexual relationship. If you are running after a man who is escaping from you, then you may be worried that you won't be able to hold on to your present lover or husband.

S

Salt

Erotic dreams of salt were said by the old dream diviners to represent semen and fertility. They may also represent your efforts to add some spice or color to a drab and neutral relationship.

Semen

Semen appears in erotic dreams in all kinds of forms and flavors, and the way in which you dream about it will often give you an insight into your sexual attitudes towards your lovers. If you dream that semen is very precious and jewel-like, then you may be a little too worshipful in the way you think about men. If you dream that it's disgusting and sickening, then your feelings have probably gone too far the other way. Dreams in which you are drinking semen are frequently in indication of your desire not only to show your lover how much you love him, but to acquire some of his sexual passion for yourself. In other words, you want to borrow some of his erotic strength so that you can love him all the more – which may show that you love him a lot, or perhaps not quite enough. If you have a sexual dream in which a man is ejaculating semen in your face, then you are adopting a classic submissive posture in your sexual relationship. Flick through a hundred porno magazines, and you will see that almost every act of sex ends with the girl receiving a faceful of sperm. Women appear to dream about the impregnating qualities of semen far more often than men, and this dream excerpt, from a 29-year-old Massachusetts girl, is an indication of how women frequently think of their entire sexual role (including pregnancy and childbirth) in erotic dreams.

I guess I was some sort of courtesan or something, because I know I was dressed in very expensive clothes, but they were also very erotic clothes as well. Gorgeous brocades and silks and jewelry, feathers and furs, but none of it covered me up. I was sitting on a settee, lying on thick cushions with a black girl fanning me. There was a strong smell of roses and lavender. The drapes opened, and my boyfriend came through. I pointed to the corner of the room, and there was a sort of small table there, with a pink glass bowl on it. He smiled, and talked very conversationally, and then he took out his cock and ejaculated into the bowl. He wiped off the last drips of sperm with a handful of rose petals, and left. After a few minutes, another man walked in. I knew his face from somewhere, but I didn't know where. He did the same thing – ejaculating into the pink glass bowl, wiping his cock and leaving. When this had happened about eight or nine times, the black girl brought over the bowl, and I had to insert a sort of rolled-up leaf into my vagina, so that the black girl could carefully pour the sperm into me. I knew that I would soon have a baby, and that the baby would have all the best qualities of all the men who had given their sperm. It seemed such a logical idea, and yet I felt very emotional and loving about the whole thing. I felt I loved all of those men, and I loved their sperm, and I was going to love the baby they had given me.

Snakes

Ever since its debut in the Garden of Eden, the snake has had phallic and sexual associations. The snake is an ancient symbol of sin and corruption – 'snake-in-the-grass' is used to describe deceivers, and liars speak, like snakes, with 'forked tongues'. But if you're making symbolic interpretations, you shouldn't forget that the snake is also a symbol of healing and regeneration. It has some magical associations, too, and some primitive cultures worshipped snakes as gods. If you have erotic dreams in which a snake or snakes appear, you may have some hidden anxiety that your lover or husband is betraying you, and doesn't feel as strongly attracted to you as you think he's pretending. You may have some repressed aversion to your lover's penis, and find that you have to overcome some squeamishness and nerves before you can handle it. Snakes represent sex without love – but sex with a cold and deadly fascination to it. Here's the dream of a 26-year-old Los Angeles girl who lived for three years with a man she disliked, but whose sexual technique and charisma she found irresistible:

I guess the idea that David was a 'snake' was planted in my mind by what my mother said about him. She couldn't stand him, and she could never understand what it was I saw in him. But he had this way of arousing your senses, of making you feel that you wanted to do crude and sexual things. I don't know what it was, this quality, but it worked on almost every young girl he ever met. I say I lived with him, but there were times when he didn't come home for nights on end. I had two or three dreams in which I *dreamed* I woke up, and there was a strange kind of slithering sensation in the bed. I lifted up the sheets to try and find out what it was, and I was just in time to see the tail of a snake disappearing down the side of the bed. Now, if I saw a snake in real life, I guess I'd run for the nearest phone and call the police or the zoo or something, but in the dream I tried to find out where it had gone. I put on my wrap, and just when I was tying my belt around my waist, I realized the snake had been lying there pretending to be the belt. It slid around my waist and around my left thigh, and I was frightened it was going to slide inside my vagina. I put my hand over my vagina so that it couldn't get in. It seemed around seven or eight feet long, and it was all cold and dry and silvery. Even though I had my hand over myself, it seemed to pour right through my fingers, and it ran its head, and about seven or eight inches of its body, right up into my vagina. It felt exactly like a penis, except that I could feel its tongue flickering in and out of its mouth, and it was tickling my womb in a way that was sexy but also very frightening. Suddenly the snake started to stiffen harder and harder, and I thought: 'Surely it's not going to come.' But then the door of the bedroom opened, and my younger sister was standing there. She was dressed in Bermuda shorts, but her breasts were bare. She has very large breasts, much bigger than mine. She stood there with her hands on her hips, watching me struggle with this snake, and really flaunting her breasts at me. She said: 'Is that all you can get – a snake? I've gone out and gotten myself a man.' I looked at the doorway again, and David was there, naked, smoking his pipe and smiling. I felt such jealousy and rage. He put his hand around my sister, and fondled her breasts. I shouted out: 'I don't even want you – all I want is my sister!' Then I woke up for real.

Your erotic dream about snakes will vary in interpretation, according to how you feel about snakes. If you have a real phobia about them, they will obviously appear in your dreams as objects of intense fear. Not all snakes that appear in erotic dreams are necessarily penises, but I don't think you'll go very far wrong if you assume they have at least some phallic role. After all, it wasn't for nothing that British slang christened the male toilet 'the snake's house'.

Soldiers

Ancient dream books used to say that if a woman dreamed of soldiers, she was being warned against casual love affairs. It's more likely, though, that you are dreaming that your husband or lover has allegiances stronger than his relationship with you. His dream uniform shows that you feel he belongs not to you but to some larger, remoter organization. It could be his career, this 'army' he belongs to. It could be nothing more complicated than the fact that he's a man, and you feel excluded from male society. If you have a sexual dream in which your lover is a soldier, you may be aroused by dominant sexual behavior from the men in your life, or you may be afraid of it. If he is battle-scarred and weary, and you dream you are making love to him and looking after him, it's possible that you see your role in his life as one of nurse and protector. Depending on the circumstances of your relationship, this may or may not be a bad thing. If you dream that you are involved in a war, and being assaulted by strange troops, your mind is expressing your natural physical fear of aggressive male sexuality.

Spectacles

If you have an erotic dream in which you find that your vision is altered or improved by wearing spectacles, you may be dreaming that your sexual relationship is not everything it seems, and that there have been several disturbing events recently which you have chosen not to recognize or accept. If you dream that you can see people without their clothes on with the aid of 'special spectacles', then you may be expressing your curiosity about sex, but your basic embarrassment and reserve about it. With 'special spectacles', you are able to observe naked people without committing yourself to an overtly sexual situation.

Storm

Just as dramatic weather conditions are used in books and movies to emphasize the emotions of the leading characters, so your dreams will sometimes provide thunder, lightning and rain to underline a passionate point. You will notice that the weather conditions in your dreams will alter according to the type of sexual relationship you are dreaming about, and that their changes are a reasonably reliable barometer to your own feelings.

T

Teeth

If you have a sexual dream in which your teeth fall out, you may be dreaming about the passing of time and the way in which you are aging and slowly losing your youthful looks. But falling teeth sometimes represent feelings of anxiety about your sexual competence or your ability to attract the men you want, and most ancient and classic interpretations link them with failure and misfortune. Calvin S. Hall suggests that dreams of dental disaster, which are very common, are a way in which the dreaming mind is expressing a feeling of guilt. Although we rarely punish ourselves *directly* in our dreams, as we do in waking life, we may dream about losing teeth or hair or part of our bodies as a symbolic self-punishment. Professor Hall quotes this dream from one of his female patients:

  I was talking with a group of people. Suddenly I heard a crunching noise and felt something drop in my mouth. I spit into my hand and saw it was a tooth. It seemed to be an eye tooth but resembled a three-legged individual salt dish. I remarked upon the oddity to my friends only to feel a sudden avalanche of falling teeth.

If this kind of disaster occurs in a sexual dream, you may be punishing yourself for some sexual failure or shortcoming. Try and recall just *when* the teeth started falling (during foreplay, during intercourse, at the point of orgasm?), and you may have a clue to the sexual hangup you feel so worried about. See also *bites*.

Telephones

It has been known for the act of telephoning, in a sexual dream, to represent the act of intercourse. But usually it symbolizes an effort to get in touch with someone you know, either literally or emotionally. A telephone bell ringing in your dream can sometimes be a reminder that you have forgotten something important, or an effort by your conscience to interrupt the sexual frolics you are dreaming about.

Television

If you have an erotic dream in which something sexual is happening on television, you may be dreaming about a love affair in which you feel physically involved, but not emotionally. If a television is switched on in the room where you dream you are making love, you may have some unconscious anxiety that your love affair is being watched or interrupted by the interference of other people.

Tools

Erotic dreams which feature tools are often fascinating insights into your own feelings about male sexuality. They can tell you a great deal about your fears and hopes, and they can also tell you what you really feel about your lover's sexual technique. Here are two dream excerpts which illustrate how two different women responded to their lovers' sexual organs in terms of mechanical tools. The first dream comes from a 29-year-old New York housewife; the second from an airline hostess from San Francisco:

I'm standing in the kitchen preparing fruit when my husband Mike walks in and says he wants to fix something. I turn around and put my arms around his neck and kiss him. He has his power drill with him, and he plugs it into the wall. He keeps kissing me and fondling my breasts, and I start to feel hot for him. He says calm down, there's plenty of time. I don't know why I should calm down, he's my husband after all, but then he tells me to stand on the kitchen chair and raise up my skirts. Well, I do that. Mike takes the power drill, and it has some kind of weird attachment on the end of it, like a metal zucchini, all covered in grease. He turns on the drill, and he pushes the metal zucchini up into my vagina. I feel this burst of pleasure, this incredible feeling, and then it's all over. He takes out the drill, packs it up, and takes off.

I dreamed I was lying in bed, and the moon was shining through the window. I knew I was going to have to get up soon and go to work. I was worried about going to work. My boyfriend Cal was asleep next to me. I put my hand on his shoulder and shook him awake. He asked me what the time was. I said: 'I don't know. The alarm clock's broken.' He sat up and said he could fix it. He climbed out of bed and walked around the room naked. I could see his penis swinging in the gloom. He came back with an optician's light strapped to his head. He pulled back the sheets and he pushed my thighs apart. He had forceps and all kinds of watchmaking stuff, and he started to pluck my clitoris with tweezers. It was exciting, but somehow it wasn't very satisfying. It was all technique and no pizzazz, if you know what I mean.

Both these tool dreams betray how these women really feel about their lovers' sexual techniques in explicit terms. The New York housewife always felt that her husband was too remote, too brutal, too quick, and that she was never satisfied. The San Francisco stewardess felt that her boyfriend was too finicky in his lovemaking, and never gave her the 'deep-down satisfaction' she felt she wanted. Some tools, of course, will have nonsexual associations. A trowel may symbolize the building of a home or a wall with which to isolate yourself. A shovel, according to one dream book, suggests that you will soon have an increase in your responsibilities. A saw may represent attempts to cut yourself off from something or somebody. But use your common sense when deciding what tools may mean. Unless they play a significant and mystical part in your dream, they probably have no ulterior meaning at all.

Transformation

When you have a sexual dream in which somebody or some object magically turns into something else, you are usually seeing the person or artifact from two different points of view. For instance, if you dream that your boss turns into a gorilla, then you are seeing him both as a boss and also as the ape your unconscious mind thinks he resembles. When clean things become dirty and people turn into beasts, you are probably dreaming out the conflict between your intellect and your lustful instincts.

— I was having sex with my husband. He was breathing hard in my ear. I looked up at him, and he was turning into a beast like a werewolf, slavering and panting as he fucked me. I dug my hands into his back, and it was dense with dirty hair. There were crusts of dried mud and excrement on his legs, and he was sweating and snorting the whole time. I didn't know whether to scream or what. I lay there petrified, with my muscles all froze up.

Trees

Trees have always had a magical significance in ancient cultures. Their shape is phallic — 'the tree of life' — but their trunks, particularly when hollow, are female. If you have an erotic dream in which a tree or trees have particular significance, you may be dreaming about a particular man's penis, or (in the case of a copse or wood or forest) many men's penises. But, more often, sexual dreams of trees have associations with the forces of life and birth and fertility. An erotic dream of trees being chopped down may be a dream of sexual conquests, or it may be a dream about your lover's sexual failure. In some occult dream books, different types of trees are interpreted as having different meanings. Aspens foreshadow loneliness, oaks are a sign of faithful love, spruce predicts good health, pines represent exciting new experiences.

Tunnels

If you have a sexual dream in which you are traveling through a tunnel, you may be dreaming about intercourse (tunnel = vagina) or you may be feeling insecure in your present situation and want to retreat from the world into a womb-like place where you have no responsibilities. Tunnel dreams can also represent confusing problems to which you are trying to find an answer ('the light at the end of the tunnel').

U

Underwear

Men seem to dream that underwear is exciting and arousing and turns them on, while women seem to dream that they have *problems* with it. Perhaps this is a reflection of how men and women feel about underwear in waking life. But whatever the reason, many women have told me about erotic dreams in which their underwear creates some kind of difficulty in the commissioning of intercourse. Sometimes the underwear is too tight, sometimes it's too voluminous and baggy. Other times it's torn or dirty or badly fitting. Dreams like these mostly seem to indicate that you have some reserve or embarrassment about exposing yourself sexually in front of a man, and that you're worried he's going to find out personal secrets about you. If you have an erotic dream in which you're wearing very exotic and erotic underwear, you're probably revealing your hidden vampishness and sensuality. The fabric of your dream underwear may tell you something about yourself. Silk and satin underwear indicates a sensuous and self-indulgent sexual personality; leather and metal indicate a strongly dominant or deeply submissive sexual personality depending on how the underwear's worn; gingham and prints indicate freshness and innocence; white indicates virginity; black indicates a love of mystery and romance. Frills and bows and ribbons have associations with a frivolous nature, and a love of teasing and coquettishness.

Urine

As Freud suggested, liquids are often interchangeable in dreams, and urine may represent semen or vaginal secretions. Some women pass a small amount of urine when they have a sexual climax, and if you're prone to this, your dreams of urinating may simply be an expression of your anxiety about it. Some sexual dreams of urination don't have anything to do with liquid at all, but represent release and relief. A Jacksonville woman said she dreamed of urination after her divorce was finally settled, and she was quite sure that the dream symbolized the letting-go of all the tension that she had felt for so long. Erotically exciting dreams of urination may indicate that you have an unconscious desire to include the sexual variation of urolagnia in your bedtime repertoire. Urolania (urinating for the sexual pleasure of it) is quite a common technique, so don't worry that you're turning into some kind of weirdo.

V

Vagina

In your erotic dreams, your vagina may sometimes represent more than just your internal sexual organ. It may represent your whole sexuality, and take on a life of its own. If your vagina performs in an unusual way in your dream, it may be showing you something important about your sexual attitudes. If it grows teeth, for instance (the mythical *vagina dentata*) and bites off your lover's penis, then it may be demonstrating how aggressive you feel towards him. You want to punish him sexually for something you think he has done to you. If your vagina talks, try and listen to what it's saying. If it hums and whistles, it may be showing you how sexually carefree you are. In one dream, a New York woman imagined that her lover kept his money, his comb and his keys in her vagina, like a billfold. She was so furious that he regarded her vagina as his property that she reached inside herself and pulled all his property out. In a dream of sexual liberation, one woman thought she could bend forward and insert her head into her own vagina. She discovered that, inside, it was more beautiful than she could have ever imagined – glistening and pink like a magical grotto. When she woke up and found that she couldn't perform this feat of double-jointedness for real, she was deeply disappointed. It is apparent that women who have made a conscious effort to realize their sexual identity dream of their vaginas in a much clearer and idiosyncratic way. As one woman said:

'I had a dream in which I saw my vagina as a *positive* thing of its own. Just the way that a tunnel is a positive statement in a mountain, or a window is a positive statement in a wall. Ask any architect. Aesthetically and functionally, there is nothing negative about an opening. I dreamed about my vagina in that positive way, and I've never thought about it as a hole, or an empty space, or a socket anymore.'

W

Womb

Because of the influence of Freudian psychology, wombs and dreams have gotten themselves intertwined in the popular imagination to the extent that any cozy hiding place is automatically considered to be a symbol of the uterus. In women's sexual dreams, however, it appears to me that wombs appear very plainly and openly, and rarely in symbolic disguises. Just as your vagina is the essence of your female sexuality, your womb is the embodiment of your ability to grow children inside you. When you have sexual dreams about your womb, you are dreaming about that ability – whether it arouses you erotically, or disturbs you emotionally, or frightens you or makes you feel proud of yourself. I like to think of dreams as forward-looking rather than retrospective. Dreams present us with future possibilities rather than anxieties about the past. So when you dream of wombs, you're dreaming of your own power to reproduce, rather than seeking the infantile security of your mother's womb, the womb you came from yourself. Here's a womb dream from a 32-year-old housewife from Los Angeles:

I was dreaming it was summer, and I was sitting in the backyard under the fruit-trees, stark naked and sipping lemonade. My hair was long and beautifully brushed, my skin was brown, my nails were polished and I felt wonderful. There was a gentle, warm breeze blowing — just enough to make my nipples stand up, but no more. I was enjoying all of this when I felt a strange sensation in my stomach. I looked down, and my belly was rising as if I was pregnant. In fact, I knew that I *was* pregnant. I leaned forward as much as I could, and I called out 'coo-ee.' There was a little gurgling chuckle inside my womb, and I knew it was a new baby. I squeezed my nose with my fingers and held my breath, so that my womb would warm up, and become a nice hot little nest for my new child.

X-Z

If you have erotic dreams about x-rays or yeggs or zircon, you're probably the best person to interpret them yourself.

As I said before, this lexicon of erotic dreams is only a prompt to help you analyze your dreams yourself. You have a knowledge of your past and your present, and you have a concept of your future, that no psychoanalyst and no dictionary could possibly hope to approach. Use this lexicon to guide you through the puzzles of the night, but do keep on adding your own opinions and your own interpretations to it. You will then begin to develop a truly personal dream dictionary, which will be an asset you can use and reuse for the rest of your life.

This book is only a small beginning in the understanding of women's erotic dreams. I wish it were possible to explore them in a book that continued for fifty times the length of this one. There is so much to discover in women's sexual personality, so many rewarding things to unearth and explore. I hope you feel, as I do, that the study of women's erotic dreams will help women everywhere to develop a fresh consciousness of their strength, their individuality, and their true role in life.

Thank you for reading, and sweet dreams.